The Consumer's Guide to Hair Transplant Surgery

Everything You Wanted To Know About Hair Transplantation

Jonathan Affleck

Author of Hair Loss Solutions

The Consumer's Guide to Hair Transplant Surgery:

Everything You Wanted To Know About Hair Transplantation

Copyright © 2015 by Jonathan Affleck

All rights reserved. No part of this publication may be reproduced in any form or by any means, including scanning, photocopying, or storing it in any medium by electronic means without prior written permission of the copyright holder.

ISBN-13: 978-1511657891

ISBN-10: 1511657898

Printed by CreateSpace

Disclaimer

This book is for information purposes only. While every attempt has been made to verify the information provided in this book, neither the author nor the publisher assumes any responsibility for errors or omissions.

The information, ideas, and suggestions in this book are not intended as a substitute for professional medical advice. Before following any suggestions contained in this book, you should consult your personal physician. Neither the author nor the publisher shall be liable or responsible for any loss or damage allegedly arising as a consequence of your use or application of any information or suggestions in this book.

About the Author

Jonathan Affleck is a hair health expert and writer. He is the author of two books: Hair Loss Solutions: Causes, Prevention and Treatments and The Consumer's Guide to Hair Transplant. He is dedicated his career to helping people understand and treat hair loss problems.

Table of Contents

Title 1
Copyright 2
Disclaimer 3
About the Author 3
Introduction 8
Benefits of Surgical Hair Restoration 11
Anatomy of Hair and Scalp 14
History of Hair Replacement Technique Developments 19
Who Are The Right Candidates for Hair Restoration Surgery? 23
Age Consideration 27
What to Do When Surgical Hair Restoration Is Not For You 29
Procedures to Avoid 31
Latest Hair Restoration Techniques 34
Female Hair Transplants 37
Realistic Hair Transplant Expectations 39
What Do I Expect After a Hair Transplant Surgery? 41
How Much Does It Cost to Get a Hair Transplant? 44
Payment Plan and Financing Options 47
Is Hair Transplant Surgery Painful? 49
How to Choose a Doctor 51
Initial Consultation 54

Hair Transplant Surgery Preparation	56
Surgery Procedure	58
How Many Hair Transplant Sessions Are Necessary?	61
Hair Transplant Surgery Methods and Follicular Units	63
Donor Area and Harvesting	68
Creating the Recipient Sites and Grafting	71
FUT	75
Follicular Unit Transplantation (FUT)	76
Important Aspects of Follicle Unit Transplantation Surgery	80
The Procedure of FUT	82
FUE	91
Follicular Unit Extraction (FUE)	92
FOX Test: Benchmark for Evaluating Candidacy for FUE	95
Surgical Procedure of FUE	97
Pros and Cons of FUE in Hair Grafting	101
Innovations in FUE	104
Comparisons between FUT and FUE	106
Robotic Hair Transplant	110
How Racial Variation Affects Hair Transplantation	113
Planning for Future Hair Loss	114
Post-Operative Care after Hair Transplant Surgery	118
Possible Side Effects and Complications	120
Caring for Your Hair after Surgery	122

When the Results of a Hair Transplant are Unsatisfactory..........125

Hair Transplant Repair...127

Other Options Available 130

Scalp Micro-Pigmentation 131

Hairline Lowering 133

Eyebrow Restoration..135

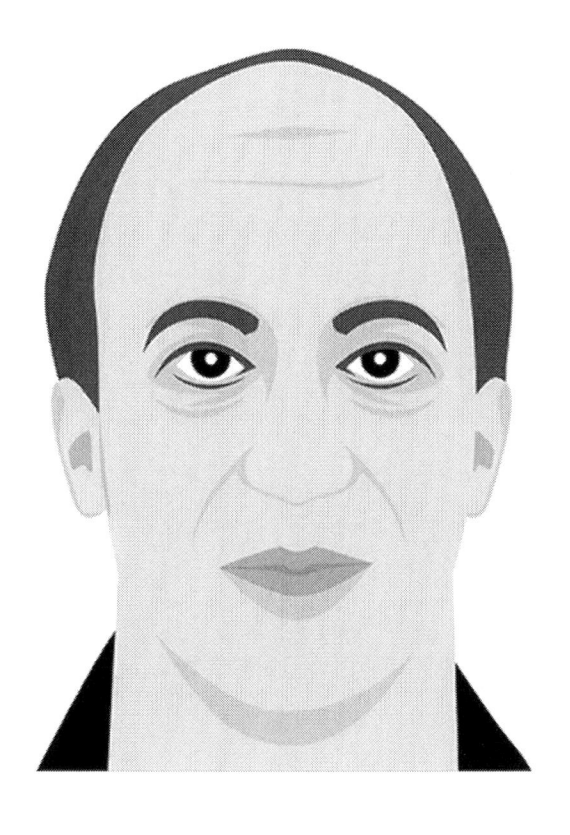

Introduction

Is it time to consider surgical treatment options for your hair loss?

Do you often wake up in the morning to find a fistful of hair on your pillow? Or do you find your bath drain clogged with lots of hair after a shower? Well, you are not alone. Hair loss is a common problem affecting faced lots of people these days.

If you are a woman, you may feel as if you are alone, but you aren't, as hair loss affects roughly 50 percent of women. It is common in men and is thought to be a sign of old age but young men are now losing hair and it is estimated that about 40 percent of men experience noticeable hair loss by the age of 35. By age 60, sixty five percent of men experience this problem. Hence, it is a common phenomenon, and if you are experiencing it, you must take comfort in the fact that you are not alone.

In spite of the statistics, some people worry about losing self-esteem when their hair is falling out all over the place. It changes your appearance, and even when you have it at a young age; it still makes you feel as if you are getting old. This is an incorrect perception because hair loss is not necessarily age related. Male and female pattern hair loss are the most common causes of the problem, but it's hard to escape the thought especially when it occurs as you are getting older.

While some people try different things to deal with hair loss from changing their hair products to taking medication, others just let it continue, opting to sit back and let nature take its course. This is the wrong approach as there are numerous hair treatments available that can help improve, if not rectify, the problem of hair loss. If you are one of those people that have tried just about all the treatments that are available, then you have most likely come across hair transplants.

Surgical hair restoration is viewed by many as a last resort when it comes to dealing with hair loss. This is because this procedure involves high financial investment and people have to undergo surgery--something that many people are uncomfortable doing. Based on the costs and the necessity of a surgical procedure, many people shun hair transplants.

If you are one of them you need to reconsider this approach as hair transplants can be quite successful, and when done correctly, are a reliable means of restoring a receding hair line or replacing hair that has been lost as a result of trauma. Even if you have tried many hair loss treatments and are tired of the whole process, it is important that you become informed about this procedure as it has been known to give great results to many men and women suffering from hair loss.

This book has all the information you need to have about hair transplants. Once you read it you know whether you are eligible for the procedure and be aware of anything you need to do to be able to get a successful hair transplant. You will find that when armed with all the information you need, it will be easy to have surgery, something that will not only restore your thinning hair, but also boost your self-esteem.

If you choose not to have surgery after all the information provided, we offer some other solutions to hair loss that you can use to deal with your problem.

Benefits of Surgical Hair Restoration

As mentioned earlier, surgical hair restoration involves moving hair from one part of the scalp to another part of the scalp that is suffering from hair loss. The hair on your head grows in groups known as follicular units that consist of two to four hairs in each group. In a case where someone is suffering from hair loss or baldness, these follicular units are transplanted to these balding areas. Some of the advantages of the procedure are:

Getting a natural look

The fact that the hair used in the transplant comes from the patient's head makes the overall effect look quite natural. The methods of transplanting hair that are used these days ensure that a natural hairline is achieved, and scars are hidden as much as possible. Once the hair grows in it is difficult, in many cases, to realize that an individual has had a hair transplant.

Restore hair on other parts of the body

Hair transplants can be done to restore hair on other parts of the body. This is helpful in the case of people who have lost hair after traumatic experiences such as being in a fire. For example, if you lose your eyebrows in such circumstances, then you can get them replaced using this procedure.

It can also be used as a cosmetic procedure for people that need to add some hair in a certain area that may not be suffering from hair loss but is still experiencing sparse hair growth. If you have had little hair growth on your eyebrow region since birth and are tired of using eyebrow pencils or tattooing your eyebrows, then this is a good procedure to use.

You are the donor

When transplanting crucial organs of the body such as kidney transplants, it is common for patients to wait for a suitable donor to be located before they can have the treatment. If a suitable donor is not found, then the procedure cannot be done. However, in the case of hair transplants, you are the donor.

No need for general anesthesia

It is common for many people to undergo hair loss surgery with their eyes open. If you are afraid of being put to sleep during surgery, then this is not a concern with this procedure. A local anesthesia is used on the area where the transplant is to be done, and you get to watch the process or engage in some other interesting activity such as watching a movie or reading a book.

Permanent results

When done by an expert, the results of hair loss surgery are permanent. As long as the problem responsible for the hair loss does not affect the hair follicles again, you can enjoy the results of your hair transplant for a long time to come. This makes it a worthwhile investment to make.

Based on these advantages, a hair restoration procedure is a good idea. However, it requires a substantial financial investment and a lot of time, so before you make the decision to have it, take time to understand the issues surrounding the procedure. Let's start with the anatomy of your hair and scalp.

Anatomy of Hair and Scalp

To understand the surgical hair restoration procedure fully, it is important to explore the makeup of your hair and scalp. This will help you to choose the right procedure for your form of hair loss as surgical hair restoration is not always the right procedure for all individuals suffering from hair loss and thinning. In addition, if you choose surgical hair restoration, understanding the anatomy of your hair and scalp will help you to understand every aspect of the procedure in terms of what will be done to your scalp during the procedure.

First you need to understand that hair does not just fall off the scalp. Normally, hair loss is caused by the action of a substance known as dihydrotestosterone also referred to as DHT on the hair follicles. This substance weakens hair follicles to a point where they are not capable of propagating healthy hair growth and any healthy hair strands fall off the scalp.

What are hair follicles?

The hair follicle is a tiny organ that is made up of special cells and structures that propagate the growth of hair strands. The growth of hair from hair follicles happens in phases. These phases are referred to as the growth phase, the cessation phase and the resting phase. These stages are scientifically known as the Anagen, Catagen and Telogen phases respectively.

Anagen   Catagen   Telogen

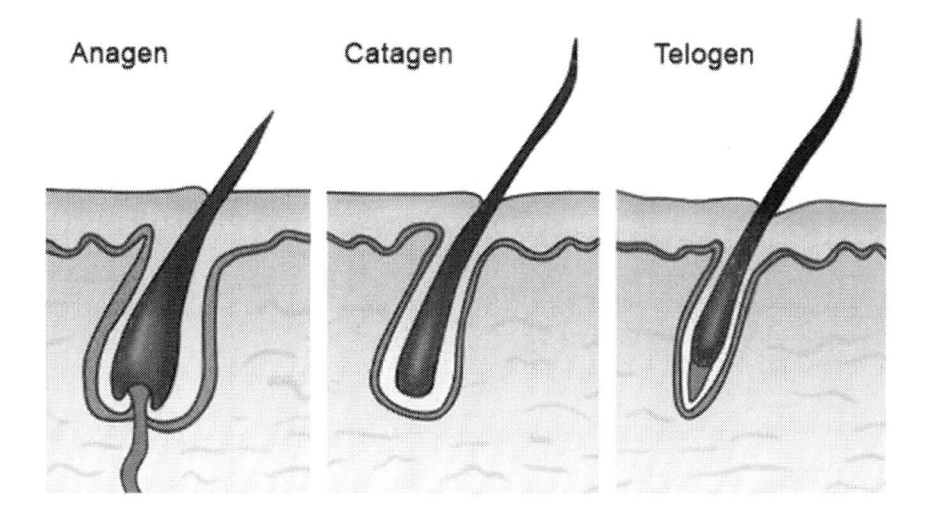

Structurally the hair follicle is made up of:

- **Papilla**: This is a large structure located at the base of the follicle that is made up of numerous connective tissues. It is a capillary loop that is important for the supply of blood to the hair follicle.

- **The matrix**: This is the other part of the hair follicle that is found around the papilla. It contains a number of epithelial cells that are known as the fastest growing cells in the human body. The cell division in this matrix produces the cells that form the main structures of hair fiber as well as the inner root sheath.

- **The root sheath**: This part of the hair follicle is made up of an inner and outer section. The root sheath protects a growing hair shaft or fiber.

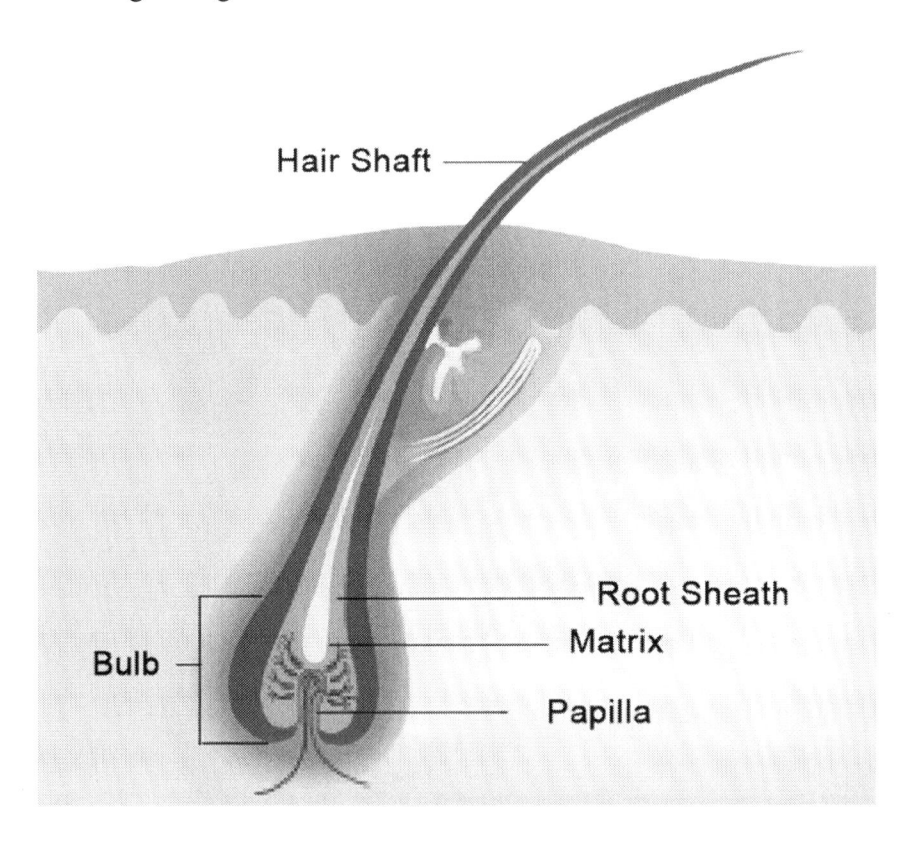

Hair fiber

Hair fiber is made up of keratin. It is horn shaped and is made up of three sections namely the cuticle, cortex and medulla. The fiber is made up of eighty percent protein, other minerals and lipids. The medulla is the innermost layer of the hair shaft. The cortex is the center part of the shaft that is responsible for strengthening and supporting the hair strands. It also provides the pigment responsible for giving the hair strand its color.

The cuticle is the outer surface of the hair shaft that protects the inner structure of the shaft. It is made up of protective transparent scale cells. The hair follicles work with the human skin to produce healthy strands of hair fiber that adhere to the three phases namely Anagen, Catagen and Telogen.

A number of issues can affect the normal hair growth cycle resulting in hair loss or hair thinning. These include taking excessively strong medication, undergoing medical procedures such as chemotherapy or radiation, hormonal changes, stress and skin ailments among others. In all these problems, apart from hormonal issues, the scalp normally recovers once the causative issue is stopped, and the hair grows back. However, in the case of hormonal interference the hair loss may continue unabated leading to bald spots and thinning hair.

The hormone responsible for hair loss in most cases is DHT or Dihydrotestosterone. This is a male hormone that is synthesized by an enzyme known as 5α-reductase in the hair follicles. This hormone causes hair loss because the hair follicles are sensitive to DHT. When they are exposed to it, they shrink, thereby losing any hair already in place and ending up completely unable to propagate new hair growth.

DHT is responsible for male pattern baldness. If left unattended, the hormone can affect all the follicles on the scalp and the hair loss will progress as it continues to affect the follicles. This is the common cause for receding hair lines. To deal with this kind of hair loss individuals are put on drugs that inhibit the production of this hormone. Once the treatment is done and the action is stopped, hair restoration surgery can be done, with the remaining healthy hairs used as the donor hairs.

History of Hair Replacement Technique Developments

Hair replacement surgery is now quite popular and has been used by many people to deal with hair loss and baldness. It has been especially useful in the case of male pattern baldness and has come a long way since it was discovered.

Early history

The first ever attempt of hair transplant surgery was performed by Diffenbach in Wurzburg, Germany in 1822. Diffenbach, a medical student, carried it out with the help of his guide Professor Dom Unger. They tried this technique on humans and animals and were somewhat successful with their experimental procedure. According to the surgical literature, few others treating baldness used Professor Unger's technique for several decades.

Modern hair transplantation started with punch technique

It was in 1930s that a dermatologist named Dr. S. Okuda in Japan first developed a new surgical method for treating loss of hair. The process involved placing thick skin flaps with hair on the hairless areas to cure hair loss on scalp, eyebrows, and even upper lips. He mostly treated patients who suffered from traumatic alopecia (loss of hair due to burns or injury). Through his punch technique, he used to pull out hair-bearing skin and implant it into small holes in the hairless areas. Once these grafts healed, growth of hair would become visible there.

All these revolutionary developments were happening during World War II. That is why this technique did not reach the western world for decades.

However, in the early 1950s, the United States saw its first successful hair transplant, which was done by Dr. Norman Orentreich on a man with male pattern baldness. The first hair transplant procedure was done for male pattern baldness by a doctor known as Norman Orentreich. He performed the procedure in New York in 1952. Unfortunately, a group of unbelieving practitioners from the medical fraternity rejected his submission of a paper detailing the procedure. However, the paper was finally published in 1959.

The demand for this cosmetic surgery kept growing during 1960s but these procedures were unable to give the desired realistic results. The professionals in this field were unable to make the surgery more effective to render a natural hair growth look. The patients ended up with a doll's head-like appearance, which made people to have negative opinions about the procedure.

However, this doctor was responsible for introducing the term donor dominance. This is a term used to describe hair that was transplanted from a donor region while continuing to exhibit the same characteristics when transplanted to bald regions. If it is a healthy, viable hair, it will continue to grow in the transplant region as it was in the donor region which eventually helps to fight baldness and thinning of hair on the scalp.

Unfortunately, even with this theory of hair dominance the grafts used in hair transplants continued to cause results that were unnatural. These grafts were 4 mm. in size which is about the width of a pencil eraser. This grafts known as plugs were excessively big because they required similar holes to be punched into the transplant region which after healing produced an unnatural look. However, for some time people suffering from hair loss or thinning chose to undergo this technique just to cover their bald spots and thinning hair regions even though the process did not guarantee optimal results.

High-resolution microscopes changed the game

Later during 1980s, a new ray of hope emerged with the new technological development. In 1984, the process of hair transplantation experienced an improvement when the technique referred to as mini grafting was introduced. This process used smaller grafts than those used before. The extracted hair-bearing strip left only a narrow scar on the donor's scalp. This strip of skin was used in small pieces of different sizes by the surgeons to give a realistic hairline. With mini-grafts, it was possible to make the implants closer together and with more hair follicles.

The scenario saw a revolutionary wave of change in the late 1980s when the use of high-resolution microscopes started taking a place in the hair restoration technique. With the help of these high-resolution mechanical supports, it was discovered that hairs grow in groups or units and not individually. This amazing fact affected a major change in performing these surgeries.

Current techniques used in hair grafting

Gradually the use of mini–micro grafts continued, overriding the use of large grafts completely. This led to the introduction of Follicular Unit Transplantation (FUT) in the 1990s. In this form of hair transplant, the idea of stereo–microscopic graft dissection came up. This involved the transplanting of naturally occurring hair grafts which required a lot of skill and care on the part of the surgeon. However, it resulted in a natural looking hair line with very good results that mimicked the natural growth of the patient's hair.

At first this form of hair transplanting was met with a lot of misgivings by experts in the sector. However after numerous successful cases it was embraced by the industry and ended up becoming quite popular. The process received further improvements as time moved on with the improvement of hair graft harvesting as well as the equipment used to do the procedure. Similarly, in 2003, a more developed extraction process also came in practice, called Follicular Unit Extraction (FUE). To this day Follicular Unit Extraction and Follicular Unit Transplantation are important in hair transplants and have resulted in great success.

Who Are The Right Candidates for Hair Restoration Surgery?

Hair restoration surgery can be of great help to people dealing with hair loss. It improves one's appearance and can lift one's self esteem immensely. Unfortunately, not everyone is eligible for this type of surgery. However, few people are aware of this as commercials and advertisements frequently shown on television and on the internet make it seem as though anyone is an ideal candidate for hair restoration surgery.

The truth is that every person is different, and it is important for each person to undergo individual analysis to ascertain whether he/she is a good candidate for the procedure. A few things are to be considered during this analysis.

- **Gender**

Hair loss in women is quite different from hair loss in men. This is because women have a diffuse form of thinning or hair loss while men have a localized form normally concentrated on the crown of the scalp. This form of surgery is only ideal for hair loss or thinning that is localized as opposed to a diffused hair loss. This is why many men find they are ideal for the surgery while few women are.

- **Extent of the hair loss**

The hair loss has to be stabilized. This is because if it is progressive, it will eventually undo the work done during the restoration surgery. For this reason, men with a class three and above hair loss measurement as measured from the Norwood scale are eligible. Anything less than this must be treated with hair loss drugs such as Propecia and Rogaine. If a patient insists on getting a transplant before the hair loss stabilizes, he/she will end up with a receding hair line positioned behind the transplanted hair which may result in an unnatural look.

- **The hair type**

People with coarse and thick hair obtain better results from this surgery, as opposed to those with fine hair. In addition, wavy hair works better as opposed to straight hair as it gives the hair more density helping to make the results of the surgery look better. This is because the coverage offered by dense and wavy hair works well when it comes to covering any scars from the surgery which is an added plus.

- **Age**

Young people suffering from hair loss are not good candidates for this procedure because it is assumed that their hair loss will likely progress further in the future. The doctor is not able to predict how bad the hair loss will eventually become, hence he /she will not know how to distribute the hairs during the transplant surgery. For such individuals, it is advisable that they fight their hair loss using drugs such as Rogaine.

- **Race**

This is based on the criteria of density. For example, in the case of Asians, they have straight hair that offers less follicular density than people of the Caucasian race. On the other hand, blacks have coarse and thick hair, which is a good characteristic for people who wish to undergo hair restoration surgery. The fact that they have dark skin also ensures that the overall appearance is much better as compared to people with light skin. There is not as much contrast between the transplanted hair and the skin on the scalp. On the other hand, they tend to have more noticeable donor scars than other races since they are prone to keloid scarring.

Caucasians that have the best results with this surgery are those with thick, coarse, dense hair and with skin color similar to their hair color. The less the contrast between the skin and the hair the better is the overall outcome.

- **Scalp Laxity**

Scalp laxity is another factor to be considered. A loose scalp is better than a tight scalp when it comes to a hair transplant because a lot of donor hair can be harvested with little scarring for the patient.

These are some of the factors that determine one's eligibility for a hair transplant. However, people that are eligible for a hair transplant also have to approach the procedure with caution as it is not a magical solution to their hair loss problem. In this way, it is important that one has a realistic idea of what can be achieved from the surgery.

It is advisable that before one considers a hair transplant he/she must ascertain that this is the only option available after having tried other mild hair loss solutions such as medication. Once you decide that you want to get a hair transplant, then ascertain that you are the right candidate for the procedure since the more suited you are for a hair transplant, the higher the chances of success. However, if surgery is not for you, there are other options available to you.

Age Consideration

At What Age Is It Right to Get a Hair Transplant?

The age at which you get a hair transplant matters, as it can determine how successful your surgery is. Generally, hair transplant specialists advise young people to approach hair surgery with caution. In fact, they recommend that a young patient consider getting a hair transplant only after they hit the age of 30.

However, there are some young patients that find this unacceptable, in which case they are advised to undergo surgery where a small number of grafts that are low in density are used. Why are they advised to do this?

Generally, hair loss replacement surgery works best when the hair loss has evened out. At this point, the surgery can be done and there will be no likelihood of the work being undone by further hair loss. If the hair loss progresses after the transplant, it means the patient will be required to go for additional surgery to deal with any patches that come up. This can be a very costly affair.

Normally, in the case of hair loss in young people, you will find that they have a receding hair line with slightly high temples. To restore such a hair line, many grafts are required so as to achieve a natural look with good hair density that can cover up any resulting scars.

If you perform a premature hair loss surgery and the hair loss progresses, then it means that you may have a bald spot forming behind the grafted hair region after the surgery, something that will result in an unnatural look. The other thing is that progressive hair loss will require further surgeries. Each time a lot of hair will be required. It is not uncommon for the donor region to be exhausted of hair so that the patient ends up with a bald spot at the back of the head. So if you do a premature hair surgery, you either run the risk of spending excess amounts of money to make the procedure an overall success or end up running out of donor hair and transferring your hair loss problem from front to back.

So what are the alternatives for young people suffering from hair loss?

Medication such as Minoxidil 5% or Finasteride 1 mg. can be used by young people for periods of six months or more instead of going for surgery. Some patients benefit from this treatment, and they experience a new growth of hair. However, this medication should be used for six months, and if no effect is registered it must be discontinued. However, while this medication is effective in some cases, it comes along with certain side effects and must be used with caution.

In a case where medication is not successful then waiting is the only option. This means that one has to wait until they get to their mid-20s and early thirties for the hair loss to stabilize. While they wait, they can use hair loss solutions such as weaves and hair systems to camouflage the problem. In addition, there are natural solutions that offer non-invasive solutions for dealing with hair loss. These include solutions like scalp massages with essential oils, using LaserCombs and using a diet that is conducive for healthy hair growth.

What to Do When Surgical Hair Restoration Is Not For You

Many people desire hair restoration surgery but, as mentioned before, not everyone is eligible for the surgery. In such cases, there is no need for despair as there are other alternatives to this form of surgery.

- **Hair loss LaserComb**

Lasers are high energy beams of light that can cut through different surfaces. In the case of hair loss and hair thinning, the LaserComb emits laser beams that penetrate the scalp tissue and enhance hair growth. Using low level lasers on the scalp is a practice that is seen as being beneficial when it comes to encouraging hair growth. These laser beams act safely on cellular compounds in the scalp that can safely promote hair growth.

While many scientists agree that laser hair combs are good for promoting hair growth, they also agree that the effects are likely to be modest and require a lot of patience on the side of the patient. In addition, it is advisable to use this form of hair loss solution on mild hair loss at a point when the hair follicles have not been excessively damaged. Hence, if you have a shiny bald spot, this is not the treatment for you.

The LaserComb is advantageous for people suffering from hair loss because it is non-invasive and can be done from home. The LaserComb is the device used for this procedure and is FDA approved, hence it is does not pose a danger to one's health, although many people believe that laser treatments are dangerous. The only side effects reported by people using the device are tingling and itching of the scalp.

- **Hair systems**

This is another solution to hair loss. These are also referred to as hair pieces. They are made out of real or synthetic hair that is put together in a form of wig that can be worn over the bald spot of a place where hair thinning occurs. They are attached either by weaving them on, clipping them on or binding them on to the scalp. Unfortunately, sometimes these hair pieces can end up looking unnatural. They also need a lot of maintenance to last for a long time.

However, when they used in the right way, they are efficient at hiding bald regions and thinning hair on the scalp.

- **Topical solutions**

This is topical or oral medication approved by the FDA for application or intake to stop hair loss and encourage healthy hair growth. Some good examples are Minoxidil and Rogaine, two topical medications that are believed to slow down and even halt hair loss in some cases. This form of medication is ideal for people that have just noticed the onset of hair loss as they can stop the hair loss in its tracks.

The other type of medication available is of an oral nature. It is known as Propecia or Finasteride. This medication stimulates hair growth as it inhibits the action of the male hormone DHT on the hair follicles which can prevent male pattern baldness.

Procedures to Avoid

If you decide to have surgery, there are some forms of hair restoration surgery that are considered outdated and that you should avoid at all costs.

You will find that some physicians are still recommending these antiquated hair restoration techniques only because they require less expertise, less staff and they don't have to use state of the art facilities for the procedure. This eventually saves them money in the long run. Here are a few examples;

- **Hair Flap procedure**

In this procedure, a flap or piece of skin with hair on it is moved from the side or back of the scalp to the front hairline. It is done to improve hairlines that have receded due to hair loss. This hair flap technique is an old type of hair loss solution. It is considered a quick solution to hair loss because it transfers a lot of hair in the least amount of time when the flap is cut off and transferred from the donor region to the area requiring the transplant.

However, this method leaves scars above and below the flap that make it look unnatural afterwards. The hair growth resulting from the transplanted flap will follow the same direction it was taking in its previous location, which means that the hair growth may look unnatural on the patient's head if the procedure is not done properly. There is also a chance that the flap's blood vessels may die off resulting in an unsightly scar for the patient. The flap could also experience infection or permanent shock that means that the section will not exhibit viable hair growth in the long run. These are a few reasons why you must avoid flap surgery.

- **Linear hair grafting**

In this form of hair loss surgery, a strip of hair measuring 3 – 4 mm. is removed from the back of the head and transplanted wholly onto the region suffering from hair loss. It requires that a small trench is cut in which to transplant the linear strips harvested from the donor region. Unfortunately, this means that the hair grows in an unnatural way that does not look good on the patient.

- **Round or square grafts**

This is another outdated form of hair transplant surgery that results in unnatural plug like grafts. Each graft is made with a hole punching device. It results in a plug of hair that is either square or circular in nature that is the size of a pencil eraser. This results in an unnatural look as the grafts do not resemble natural hair growth in any way. They are too big, which compromises blood flow and often results in a lack of hair growth in the mid-section of the graft. The resulting look is similar to doll hair, something that is unattractive on patients.

Recently there has been a development of mini and micro grafts that are smaller in size than the pencil sized ones. They still result in an unnatural look, and for this reason this kind of procedure is normally passed over in favor of those using follicular units. These units are made up of 1-4 hair strands that provide a look that is natural in the long run.

- **Scalp reduction**

It is also called Alopecia Reduction, Male Pattern Reduction or Galeoplasty. This involves the cutting away of the bald part at the top of the head after which the edges of the nearby hair bearing skin are stretched forward phasing off the bald spot. This procedure results in bad scars and can result in accelerated hair loss due to shock. It also results in an unnatural looking hair line as the direction of hair growth is altered as well as hemorrhaging, among other negative results.

Latest Hair Restoration Techniques

Hair restoration has come a long way, and there is no need to invest in techniques such as hair flap and linear hair grafting, among others, that are outdated. The fact is that hair restoration is still quite popular because many people are dealing with hair loss issues resulting from disease, age and scarring as a result of trauma. If you are dealing with hair loss and want to do something to turn it around then consider one of these modern hair restoration techniques.

Modern hair restoration techniques

The modern hair restoration techniques are based on an idea introduced by Dr. Bernstein, known as Follicular Transplantation. Based on this concept, the results of modern day hair transplants look quite natural.

- **Follicular Unit Transplantation (FUT)**

Follicular transplantation is when hair is transplanted in naturally occurring follicular units known as grafts. The grafts are made up of 1 – 4 hair strands harvested from the donor region, which is the place with healthy hair strands unaffected by the issue resulting causing the hair loss.

Once these hairs are harvested, they are grafted into needle sized holes which are referred to as recipient sites that are cut into the balding area. Once the surgery is successful, the transplanted hair follicles begin producing new hair growth after two to three months. In a year's time, with a successful surgery, the hair transplant will be fully grown in, meaning it will be fully merged into the scalp.

- **Follicular Unit Extraction (FUE)**

In this form of follicular hair restoration, the grafts are harvested singly. This means they are harvested one by one from the back or side of the scalp based on where the hair is most dense on the scalp. Tiny recipient sites are cut into the bald section into which the grafts are inserted. The donor wounds that form when the donor hair is harvested heal completely after about ten days.

This process is quite different from Follicular Unit Transplants based on how the follicles are harvested. In FUT, the follicular units are harvested in a thin long strip as opposed to when it is done follicle by follicle as in the case of FUE. In both cases, when successful transplants are done, the follicles blend in well, and healthy hair starts growing from them thereby taking care of the hair loss issue. The only difference is in the appearance of the grafts. These two modern hair restoration techniques are ideal for people whose hair loss has stabilized.

- **Robotic hair restoration**

This is an improvement on the follicular transplantation procedures, and it involves the automation of these hair restoration surgeries. The use of automation enhances the procedure in many ways. It uses image guided robots to separate the follicular units needed for the grafting, which guarantees precision and minimizes damage to the hair follicles. It also reduces harvesting time and increases the chances of the grafts being viable. All these things guarantee a successful operation that offers better results as compared to those done without robotics.

Female Hair Transplants

Hair transplants are recommended for about 90 percent of the cases of baldness diagnosed by doctors. For this reason many women dealing with hair loss think that they can use this kind of hair treatment to deal with their hair loss. This is not the case.

The reason why hair transplants work in a lot of male hair loss cases is because hair loss in men is normally localized. Most of the time it occurs on the crown. In women, very few cases are localized as many of them experience diffuse hair loss.

Diffuse hair loss is when hair is lost in different sections of the scalp which results in bald patch formations all over the head where the hair has fallen or thinned out. This makes it hard to find healthy sections of hair with viable hair strands. In men, the sides and back are full of healthy hair, which makes them ideal sites for harvesting hair to be transplanted on the bald spots. In women, most of the hair on the scalp is infected. If these infected hair follicles are transplanted to the bald spots on a woman's head, they will just end up falling out. No healthy hair growth will be experienced, meaning the surgery will be a failure and a waste of money.

The other factor that prevents women from using hair transplant surgery is the formation of their frontal hairline. In men, the hairline is often receding which is a form of hair loss that can easily be dealt with by undergoing hair transplant surgery. With women, their hair loss rarely affects their hair lines, so they don't have to get transplant surgery to deal with it. Women are usually concerned mostly with the loss of volume that happens with their hair loss. Surgical hair restoration does not do much to increase volume, hence many of them cannot use it as a solution to hair loss.

Having said this, a small percentage of women are good candidates for surgical hair transplants. This percentage is made up of:

- Women that have lost hair as a result of trauma, such as in the case of traction alopecia.
- Women who have had some cosmetic surgery before, that may have ended up causing hair loss around the incisions made during the cosmetic surgery. Such women can have hair transplanted onto the scars to hide the scars.
- Women that have suffered from a form of pattern baldness that is similar to male pattern baldness. Such cases include vertex thinning of hair and hairline recession.
- Women suffering from Alopecia Marginalis, which is similar to traction alopecia.
- Women that have lost hair due to trauma from scarring, chemical burns or scars caused by fire burns.

If you are suffering from hair loss, then check to see if you are a successful candidate for the procedure by looking at the above pointers. You can also get a consultation from a qualified hair specialist. If you find that you are not a good candidate for the procedure, then explore other ways of dealing with your hair loss. This will prevent you from wasting time and money and ultimate disappointment.

Realistic Hair Transplant Expectations

The point of hair transplant surgery for many people is basically cosmetic, the patient wants to improve his/her appearance and get rid of the bald spots that give him/her a funny appearance and bring down his/her self-esteem.

Unfortunately, some patients view transplant surgery as a magical solution that will restore their hair line to what it used to be before the hair loss occurred and end up with disappointment once the hair replacement surgery is done. There are limitations depending on many factors. Things to consider in order to get a realistic picture of the result to expect from this surgery include:

Age

If you are a victim of male pattern baldness and get the surgery when you are in your late thirties to forties, you cannot expect your hair to be restored to look like that of a 20 year old. This surgery is not to make you look younger rather, it is done to restore your hairline. If you end up looking younger as a result, it is just a bonus.

Possible future hair loss

It is important to know that there is a likelihood that your hair loss will progress and will require additional surgery to deal with the issue. Hair loss surgery is not a procedure that stops hair loss. It is used to cosmetically replace hair to sections where the hair has been lost. For this reason, it is important that, as a patient, you are aware of the need for future additional surgeries to deal with any additional hair loss and the costs of these surgeries as well. In addition, you need to be made aware of the importance of safeguarding the healthy hair in your donor region in case you need additional surgery in the future.

Heredity

Some people have a history of hair loss in their family and this can be used to make a rough estimate of the extent of hair loss to expect. This will help you to know the amount of donor hair you may need and the age at which you should have the surgery in the first place.

The type of hair

Your hair type also influences the success of hair loss surgery in a big way. This refers to the texture of the hair, color and whether it is wavy or straight. These aspects will determine the success of the hair transplant surgery in terms of the overall look. The denser the hair the better that the donor hair will cover the bald spot. It will also help to hide any scars resulting from the procedure.

The health of the patient

This procedure requires a patient to be put under anesthesia, and it takes a couple of hours based on the extent of the hair loss. This means that a patient will be required to be quite healthy to withstand the surgery and also end up with a successful result.

The cost

This surgery is not cheap, and it gets more expensive the more pronounced the hair loss is in a patient. This aspect must be clearly outlined to the patient and everything done to ensure that it is a success. This includes a thorough pre-analysis of the patient's hair loss and a selection of the right way to undergo surgery. The doctor expected to do the surgery must also have a track record of carrying out successful procedures as well. This will assure you of expert guidance and good results.

By considering these points, you will be able to make the right choice when it comes to hair loss surgery.

What Do I Expect After a Hair Transplant Surgery?

Many commercials advertising hair transplant surgery give an unrealistic picture to patients. Some promise exceptionally good results, while others say that you can have the surgery and get back on your feet ready to get back to work the next day.

These are unrealistic ideas. First, you need to know that hair loss surgery is a serious procedure that will require some preparation and adequate recovery time. In terms of the success of the implants and when to expect new hair growth, it also requires patience on the side of the patient and an adherence to the doctor's advice on how to treat the transplant region. If done properly, the results of a hair transplant surgery are permanent. Based on the following outline, you can see what to expect after a surgery. This will give you a realistic picture of the results you can expect to get.

The day after the surgery you can expect some soreness and numbness on the donor region as the healing starts to occur. You will be expected to wash the transplanted area properly and ensure that there is no blood in the region.

Three days after the surgery the numbness and soreness in the donor region will begin to reduce and any scabbing on the transplanted region will be gone. You can expect some redness and swelling on the scalp.

A week later, the redness and swelling will be gone from the transplant region. The soreness and numbness will also disappear from the donor region. After a fortnight, if the hair transplant surgery is a success, hair will begin to sprout on the transplant region that will look like a 4 day old beard. In the donor region, sutures resulting from the surgery will start to heal, and any numbness or soreness will be completely gone.

In the period following the two weeks, right up to the eighth week, there will be some shedding from the transplant region as the hair follicles drop off old hair and enter into a dormant stage. Do not be alarmed as this is just the hair follicles functioning in their normal way. The sutures are removed and any knots at the region where the sutures were will fall off as the region heals.

In three to six months, the transplant region will begin to sprout fresh hair that will be quite fine at first. The donor region will be completely healed with no discomfort. The growth in the transplant region will continue to become strong. Generally at eight months most hair transplant beneficiaries have a growth of hair sprouting from the transplant region that can be groomed, although it appears thinner than the other regions of the head. However, as it continues to grow it thickens.

It is advisable that you make frequent visits to the surgeon after hair loss surgery to ensure that all is progressing as required. You will be able to ascertain that you are treating the transplant region and donor regions in the right manner to avoid interfering with the results of the surgery. This will also allow the doctor to see whether a second procedure is required to improve the results. Generally in two years, the full results of the surgery will be evident.

How Much Does It Cost to Get a Hair Transplant?

The cost of hair transplants is a factor that prevents many from using this solution when dealing with hair loss issues. While these procedures can be quite costly, you do get value for money. The techniques used in hair transplant surgery have come a long way from some of the crude methods used in the past such as the flap procedure. This means that you can be guaranteed of good results. Since a good transplant can last a lifetime, it is a worthwhile investment.

The cost of hair transplant surgery differs from case to case. This means that the extent of your hair loss has to be considered. The greater the hair loss, the more money you need to spend to get the results you want.

The cost of a hair loss transplant session is calculated based on the number of grafts to be surgically harvested and transplanted onto the section suffering from hair loss. It also depends on the length of time it takes to transplant the grafts. This refers to how long it will take to harvest the grafts from the donor region and successfully set them into the transplant region.

As outlined in the previous section, the technique you choose will also determine the cost of the surgery. This is in terms of the use of follicular units as compared to micro grafting. The use of follicular units requires more precision as compared to what is done when using micro grafting; hence it is more expensive to use follicular units. However, the use of follicular grafts yields better results than what is achieved when using micro grafting; hence it is worth the extra costs for anyone looking for perfect results.

In addition to this, the timing of the surgery matters because if you undergo surgery when your hair loss has not dissipated, you will require follow up surgery for future hair loss. For this reason, getting the surgery done at the right time will lead to excellent results with no need for follow-up surgery, something that will reduce the overall cost of keeping your hairline intact.

Although the cost of your hair surgery will be based on the number of grafts to be transplanted, generally hair replacement surgery costs between $4000 and $15,000. To get an accurate figure, you can calculate the cost of a hair transplant based on the grafts you will get transplanted. Prices normally stand at $3 - $8 per graft, with $5 - $6 being the average cost per graft. The price per graft usually drops as a sort of discount for the patient, as the size of the surgery increases. Unfortunately, this procedure is rarely covered by insurance.

However, all things considered, hair loss surgery is a cost-effective solution as compared to other ways of dealing with hair loss such as the use of hair systems and other solutions such as weaves and wigs in women. The amount you spend on these solutions calculated in the long term cannot compare to the cost of a hair replacement surgery which, when done correctly, produces long lasting results.

When the right research is done, and the right experts are used, the cost of this surgery is worth it in the end. Many people have successfully recovered their hairline by using this procedure. It is hard to tell that they suffered from hair loss in the first place. The important thing is to take time to look around and identify the right expert who will ensure that any money you use is well spent and who gives you the results you desire. This is not a medical procedure where costs can be cut, as you will ultimately be cutting down on the excellent results you can expect to get from it.

Payment Plan and Financing Options

Hair transplant surgery is not a cheap medical procedure, and the costs increase with the amount of care and expertise applied. The exact number of grafts required and the amount of necessary work depends upon the individual. First of all, you will need to have a consultation to find out whether hair transplant surgery is the best option for you and how much it is going to cost to get your hair looking the way you would like.

Because you want a successful procedure with natural looking results, you need to find an experienced expert. Some cheap options may end up costing you more later. A quality procedure is going to save you money in the long run. This does not mean, however, that it is beyond the ordinary person's budget.

Hair transplant surgery is not covered by medical insurance, but you do not have to save the entire cost. In fact, there are a number of financing options available for you, and many hair transplant clinics will be able to help you by offering a reasonable payment plan so you can space out the payments.

Affordable monthly payments are a great option if you are on a tight budget and cannot pay a lump sum. Many hair replacement clinics will accommodate you with a financing solution. You need to ask during your initial consultation. The conditions of the payment plan will be discussed upfront. The monthly payment rates vary between lenders and they are based on the terms you apply for, your credit standing and, of course, the total amount financed.

Some institutions might refer you to a third-party credit agency, and these allow qualifying customers to borrow money, which they will pay back over time with interest until the full amount, agreed upon has been repaid. If you choose this form of credit you will have a longer period to pay the money back. You may choose 24, 36 or 48 months, depending upon how much you can afford to repay per month. The longer the repayment period, the higher the interest rate will be.

Another option is to use your credit card to pay for your hair transplant surgery, but bear in mind credit card companies are going to charge a high interest rate, so you will probably get a better deal using the credit facilities offered by the hair restoration expert. Credit card companies have promotional offers from time to time though, so it is always worth investigating. You will need to consult with the clinic official first, to find out what kind of payment plans, if any, they offer. You might also be able to negotiate the cost and get a better rate or longer repayment period. You can make the best decision after you look at all your options.

If you choose a credit plan, you need to make sure the payment plan is manageable. Overestimating how much you can afford to pay back each month is a huge mistake, so be sure to choose an installment plan that works for you. That way you will be able to afford the hair transplant surgery you really want.

Is Hair Transplant Surgery Painful?

One of the things that people often ask when considering hair transplant surgery is whether the surgery will be painful or not, they also want to know if they will have the option of anesthesia. The scalp is quite sensitive, and since hair restoration surgery requires skin cutting as the hair is harvested from the donor region and during transplantation of the hair, you can expect a bit of pain.

However, there is nothing to be afraid of as it is not debilitating pain. Many people describe the pain they feel during hair transplant surgery as bearable. One of the times you can expect to feel pain during the transplant is when your scalp is injected with anesthetic before the procedure commences. This is done to ensure that the section on which the surgery will be carried out is numb throughout the process in order to keep you from feeling any pain. Otherwise it would be a very uncomfortable procedure.

Once the transplant is complete and the anesthesia wears off, you can expect the region to feel a bit tender. There may be a little pain and swelling, but it will go down within a couple of days as the effects of the operation wear off.

The modern form of hair loss surgery is a world away from the procedures that were used in the past. The technology has improved, specialists have improved their skills, and there is more medication available to deal with pain issues. For these reasons, you can expect the surgery to be bearable even with a little pain.

It is important to choose an experienced surgeon with access to modern tools in a well-equipped practice. They should also have competent support staff. This kind of set up requires money to maintain, so such surgeons will not be inexpensive. But you will be sure that they are doing expert work and as a result of their expertise, any pain will be minimal and the recovery period will be shortened. The outcome of the surgery will also be to your satisfaction.

Some people are afraid of surgery and have a very low pain threshold. In such cases the patient may be mildly sedated throughout the surgery. This helps them to get through any pain that they might experience and also allows surgeons to do their work in peace.

After surgery, it is common for specialists to give their patients mild pain killers to help combat any pain they may feel before the scalp heals. They also give mild sedatives that the patient can use to ensure that they get a good night's sleep- rest is quite important for a quick recovery. The mild discomfort you may experience does not compare to the results that you are likely to get from successful hair restoration surgery. For this reason, many people have had hair transplants and many more will continue to do so.

How to Choose a Doctor

As described before, the doctor or surgeon you use for your hair restoration surgery does not only determine the results you get but the way that you heal afterwards. For this reason, it is important to take to the time to choose the right doctor.

When looking for a doctor to do a hair restoration surgery, one has to consider the following:

Find a recognized doctor

This means that you need to get a doctor that is registered with a trusted consumer organization which carefully screens doctors based on their skills and ethics. A good example of such an organization is the Alliance of Hair Restoration Surgeons. From their database, you will be able to get information on a number of experienced surgeons in your area. You can then narrow them down to the one that appeals to you.

In addition, you can contact your state medical board to determine that no surgeon you have selected has complaints made against them for unethical behavior or for carrying out botched hair transplants in the past.

Carefully screen the doctors

Once you select a few surgeons from the pool of the many that are available, you will need to visit each of them and get a feel for how they work and whether they will meet your expectations. This will require you to see their practice in person, question the kind of team they work with and how long they have been working together, and ask for references from people that have undergone successful surgery with them.

If possible, visit one of these patients in person just to have an idea of the kind of results you can expect. The doctor has to have a well-equipped practice that you are sure will meet all your needs in the case of any eventuality. In addition, in the case of any complications, you need to know that they will handle you with care and ensure that you make it through the surgery in one piece.

It is advisable to choose small practices that are well equipped and have a low staff turnover as well as a good track record when it comes to successful surgeries. These normally have a track record of giving better services, as opposed to large establishments.

Get references

Before making your decision, you may ask the names and phone numbers of patients that have undergone a successful surgery with the doctor of your choice. Obtain before and after pictures of the patients so that you can determine the skills that the doctor has and get an idea of what to expect.

The pictures must be taken from the same angle, with the same background and lighting. Ensure that the references you obtain belong to patients that were dealing with the kind of hair loss with which you are dealing. They should also have similar hair types because this will help you know what you can expect from the surgery.

Interview the doctor and the technical staff

Lastly, attend a one-on-one session with the doctor who will be performing your surgery. The references that you have obtained have to be for work done by him/her so that you are sure that you are using the right expert. Some doctors send technicians to work on potential patients even after they conduct a consultation in person. Make sure that the doctor and technical staff you talk to are the same individuals that will be performing your surgery. Ensure during the interview that the experts satisfy your curiosity.

Initial Consultation

Having an in depth consultation with your doctor is important before you settle on a date for the operation. You need to be sure that you are dealing with someone who is aware of what they are doing. You need a professional with a competent team that has performed successful surgeries countless times before and with evidence to prove it.

To ensure that you get the right doctor, do not be afraid to ask a lot of questions. If you come across a doctor who is unwilling to answer your questions, then that may not be the right doctor for you.

The questions you ask during a consultation should revolve around the doctor's experience, the kind of hair transplants they do and the kind of after surgery support they can offer you until you are properly healed. By the time you sit down for a consultation, you should have assured their experience by checking their reputation, references and talking to patients who have undergone surgery in their practice successfully.

When you sit down with them, first address the current state of hair loss you are experiencing. This means you have to address whether you are the right candidate for a transplant.

If you find that you are eligible for hair loss surgery, the next thing is to ask how much hair you will need to cover the region suffering from hair loss. This will depend on the size of your bald spot and the hair density you want to achieve from the surgery.

Also, you need to know if you have enough hair in your donor region to cover the bald spot. This will ensure that you have a realistic picture of the results you are going to get after the surgery. In some cases, the baldness is so extensive, and the donor hairs are so few that it is an exercise in futility to undergo a transplant. In such cases, other options have to be considered for you. A good doctor will be open with you during the consultation and let you know where you stand.

If you are a viable candidate for a hair transplant, the next issue to address is cost. You also need to know how long the procedure will take and how long you have to wait to see the results of the surgery. When it comes to cost, you can also ask if they offer payment plans as this will help you to meet the costs of the surgery.

Find out the length of time that the procedure will take, including the recovery period so you can better organize work and family commitments to ensure you have the necessary time at hand to undergo the procedure.

You also need to ask about post-op care and be aware of how many checkups you will need from the doctor as he/she checks to see that everything is progressing well after the surgery. You need to have access to your doctor after the surgery so that he can help you be at ease about the recovery experiences you are likely having and to be sure that all questions you have about the healing process are answered.

Hair Transplant Surgery Preparation

Once you do enough research and are familiar with the aspects surrounding hair loss surgery, you may decide to undergo it. If you do, then you need to know how to prepare yourself for this procedure. Like any other surgical procedure, you cannot just get up and go to the hospital. You need to be prepared in advance as it will help the procedure to be successful.

Preparation for hair loss replacement surgery normally starts three weeks before the procedure. During this time, the patient is asked to stop taking any medication that may interfere with the surgery. In this group are supplements, medication and/or vitamins that can make you bleed excessively during the surgery. This includes prescription and over-the-counter medications such as Advil, aspirin and Coumadin, among others.

Vitamins and supplements such as Vitamin E, garlic supplements, Echinacea, fish oil and Gingko Biloba are avoided because they can also make you bleed. Some of these vitamins and supplements are considered to be safe, and it would never occur to some people to stop taking them in lieu of impending hair replacement surgery. This is why it is important to disclose to your doctor every vitamin, supplement, herb or medication that you are taking so that you can get advice on the ones to avoid and the ones to keep. One vitamin you will be encouraged to take starting about two weeks before the surgery and be expected to continue taking for two weeks after the surgery is Vitamin C. This is recommended in order to help with healing.

Some other things that you must avoid are nicotine and alcohol, which may interfere with your healing and the success of the procedure. Patients are also advised to avoid staying too long in the sun to keep the scalp from getting sunburnt, which may cause it to be tender and make it difficult to do the procedure.

If you have chosen an experienced and conscientious doctor, then he/she will make sure that you are frequently contacted by the staff as the surgery day approaches. This is to ensure that you are following the doctor's instructions and maintaining a lifestyle that will optimize the success of the surgery. Once the transplant day arrives, you will be asked not to eat or drink anything after midnight on the night before you have to go for the transplant procedure; this includes water. There is no need to feel deprived, as after the hair transplant procedure begins patients are normally provided with breakfast and lunch.

On the day of the procedure, patients are advised to avoid applying any hair products on the scalp. This means that you should avoid any hair sprays, hair gels and conditioners. It is also important to wear loose clothing that you can easily pull off and put on before and after the surgery. If you will be requiring oral sedation, then make sure you have a designated driver to get you home after the surgery. If you decide to have only the area on which the surgery is being done numbed, then you can bring a book, a video or some of your favorite music to listen to during the surgery to keep you from focusing too much on the surgery as it progresses.

Surgery Procedure

Make sure you know exactly what will happen on the day of your procedure. You need to get a step by step information on what you will go through: from the time you arrive at the hospital to the time when you are discharged. This will make you feel at ease and also help you to prepare for any eventuality. Normally, hair transplant surgery involves the following;

Arrival

When you arrive at the hospital you will be expected to fill out some forms with important details needed by your doctor. After this, you will be checked to ensure that you are physically fit for the procedure. This involves checking your blood pressure and some other necessary medical checks.

Briefing

Once you are deemed to be fit for the procedure, you will be wheeled into a hair transplant procedure room. The doctor will go over your expectations for the surgery and also explain what they are planning to do to you throughout the surgery. This is to ensure that you have an idea of what you will undergo to put you at ease.

Anesthesia and harvesting

This will be followed by an anesthesia injection in the donor region. This will make the area numb and ensure that you do not feel any pain. The doctor will then remove strips of your hair tissue. At this time, you will be lying face down on the operating table. The procedure will go on for 30to 45 minutes based on the amount of hair that you need to cover the transplant section.

Preparation of harvested hair into required grafts for transplanting

Once the hair is harvested, the doctor will seal up the donor site and hand over the harvested strips to technicians so that they can separate them into follicular units for use during your surgery. These units are dissected using a microscope into units of 1 – 4 hair strands.

Normally after the hair is harvested there is a break during which the procedure room and tools for the second phase of the transplant are prepared. At this time, you can take a restroom break and walk around.

Grafting

The second phase of the surgery will involve grafting the harvested hair strands into the transplant region. The doctor will prepare the recipient sites by cutting tiny incisions into the transplant region. It is in these incisions that the donor hair will be implanted.

The doctor will try to mimic the alignment and distribution of hair as it occurs on the rest of the scalp. Once the incisions are made, technicians will proceed to place the grafts into the incisions in the correct direction. This will continue until the donor hairs are finished and the proposed transplant region is covered as planned. This procedure requires a lot of time and care.

Post operation pack

Once the procedure is done, you will be given some antibiotics, mild pain relievers and anything else necessary for your care after the surgery. You may choose to spend the first night in the facility, but many people are able to go home the same day and continue recovery from home. This is followed by frequent consultations with the physician as healing continues to make sure that all is working out as intended.

Many people think that they can leave the operation table and be at work the next day. It is important that you schedule enough time for your operation and the recovery period, during which you cannot undergo strenuous activities. This will ensure that you heal properly and the operation is successful.

How Many Hair Transplant Sessions Are Necessary?

Once you consider having hair transplant surgery, you may want to know how many transplant sessions will be required to deal with your hair loss. The answer is not simple; many factors must be considered.

Determining factors include the extent of your hair loss, the number of implants required per hair restoration surgery, the desired density, and the type of procedure. Other factors include the color and quality of the donor hair, scalp laxity, donor hair density, and facial features. At times, it is recommended to schedule two or more sessions. For instance, a decent-looking hairline can be achieved in just one hair restoration session, but the hair density and refinement most people desire usually requires two or three sessions.

You may need only one session if you require less coverage; other clients may need one or two sessions to treat the entire frontal hair area, as well as midscalp and/or the bald spot on the top of the head.

Typically up to 5,000 follicular units can be harvested for hair transplant, but this does not mean that all these hair follicles should be grafted in a single session. In fact many hair transplant institutes harvest only 2,000 grafts in one surgical session within 24 hours. Depending on the patient's preferences, sessions can be scheduled over a period of time.

Additionally, more sessions may be necessary to fill in "spaces." The timing of these additional sessions would depend, of course, on the needs of each patient as well as the progression rate of the loss of his/her remaining natural hair. Generally, though, sessions are spaced at least three months apart (minimum) in order to allot time for establishing new grafts and the head's blood supply.

And most importantly, the total number of sessions will be determined by your expectations. How much improvement do you want to achieve after your transplant? You need to be realistic as results will depend on the current extent of your hair loss. Your expectations should not ignore the current level of your hair loss, which will determine the number of necessary sessions to achieve the desired results. For example, if your hair loss is extensive and there's not much supply of donor hair, then you cannot expect a full head of transplanted hair. The supply of your donor hair and the extent of your hair loss in such a case will result in few hair transplant sessions since there is not much donor hair.

Hair Transplant Surgery Methods and Follicular Units

Hair transplant surgery has come a long way since its invention in Japan. Currently, Follicular Unit Transplantation (FUT) and Follicular Unit Extraction (FUE) are the two major methods used for providing a new patch of healthy hair for a bald area. Both hair transplantation techniques are known for their ability to provide natural looking hair with no signs of surgery.

Hair transplantation techniques: FUT & FUE

FUT is performed by a strip technique where the back of the head, which generally has a larger amount of natural hair, is chosen as the donor area. A patch of scalp that has the highest number of hair follicles is removed from the area and used for transplantation. Alternatively, in the FUE method, the surgeon extracts hair follicles individually and then uses them for transplantation.

FUE and FUT use small groups of hair consisting of 1 to 4 natural hairs for the procedures. These groups are called Follicular Units (FUs). The entire transplantation process is completed using these follicular units. Hence, no artificial material is used in any way.

When choosing follicular units, surgeons look for the best type of hair roots for quality hair. They focus on the backside of the head. The hair roots on the backside of the head are naturally stronger and are less prone to thinning compared to the hair at the front. These roots do not become inactive, even during hormonal changes in the body. Selection of healthy hair follicles plays an important role because these roots, after being transplanted, are expected to grow natural hair.

Follicular Units

Finding follicular units has brought about a revolutionary change in hair transplantation technology. Previously, it was understood that the growth of scalp hair happens as single strands. However, the truth is that hair grows in small clumps with between 1 and 4 strands. These groups of scalp hair are called Follicular Units. The presence of follicular units on the scalp is not detectable with the naked eye. The groups of hair become visible when the hair length is cut down to leave only 1 mm on the scalp. When using an instrument called a densitometer which allows a profound magnification of 30x, the units can be seen effortlessly.

Structure of follicular units

The composition of a follicular unit is interesting. When looked at closely, you will find not just hair follicles, but also blood vessels and nerves. A small muscle called erector pilorum is also part of the unit. This muscle is actually what makes a feline's hair stand erect on its ends when the animal is faced with a threat and intends to scare the adversary away by increasing its size via its hair standing straight up. The follicular unit is covered with collagen that lends it a unique appearance.

These units are independent structures, complete in their formation, which play an unparalleled role in hair growth on the scalp. That is why during transplantation, it is important that these units be handled very carefully without causing any damage to any part to generate successful results.

Follicular units are placed very close to each other covering the smallest possible zones on the scalp. This allows a greater amount of transplants to be done in the available space. Moreover, since follicular units are reflective of the way hair grows naturally, the effect of the transplantation is very natural and appealing.

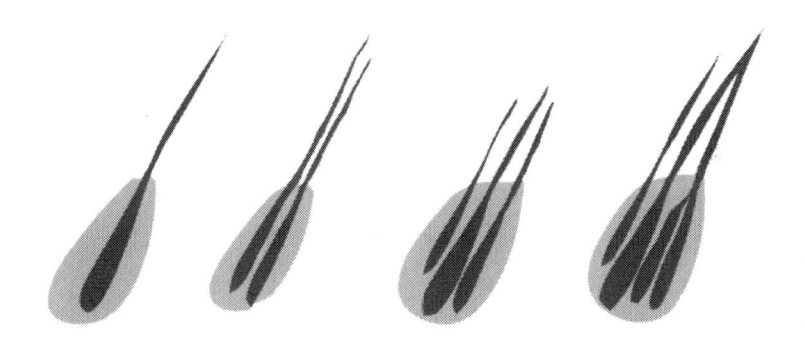

How are follicular units preserved in FUT and FUE?

In both techniques, the preservations of follicular units are handled with the utmost care. These FUs are required to stay alive until transplantation. After the extraction, follicular units are preserved in an environment that is similar to the condition of the human body. While being worked on, the follicles are kept in a moist environment which lowers their mortality rate.

Follicular units collected under the FUE method are more prone to die. This is because the FUE method gather hair follicles independently, which leaves a little of the protective tissue at the base. If a hair follicle suffers damage because of bad preservation, it could result in a poor growth rate and bad quality of hair. Hence, the success rate of hair transplantation largely depends on the way the follicular units are preserved.

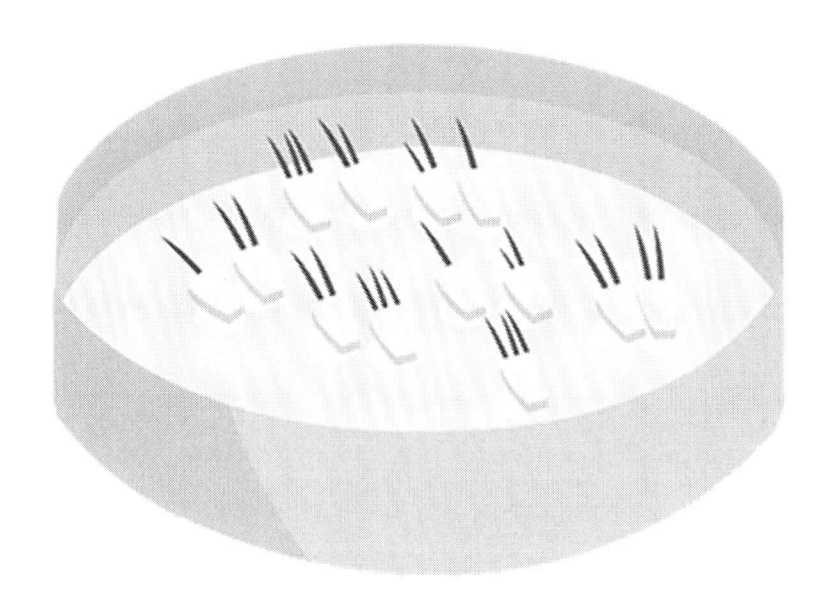

How many follicular units are required for a transplantation procedure?

In general, 1,000 to 5,000 follicular units are required for a complete transplantation. The surgeon may need more, in case there is a greater area of the head that is bald. With proper pre-transplantation care and careful transplantation, using either of the above techniques, a good density ranging from 30 to 90 follicular units per cm^2 can be attained.

Donor Area and Harvesting

The donor area is the section from which hair grafts to be used for hair transplant surgery are taken. This is a part of the scalp with hair that is unaffected by the problem causing hair loss in an individual. In men suffering from male pattern baldness, the donor area is normally at the back or sides of the scalp. This hair is harvested with the hair follicle intact and transplanted to the area suffering from hair loss, where, if it is successful, it will grow in a year's time to maturity, thereby covering the bald spot and restoring one's hairline.

The issue of hair harvesting for hair transplant surgery sounds simple, but it involves quite a few issues. First of all, there are a couple of techniques used to harvest hair from the donor area. Regardless of the technique used to harvest the hair, the result must be that the hair harvested is viable, which means it is healthy and will grow strongly after the surgery. The second thing is to ensure that it is harvested at an angle that corresponds with the tissue in the transplant region. Some of the techniques used to harvest donor hair include FUT strip excision harvesting and FUT follicular unit extraction.

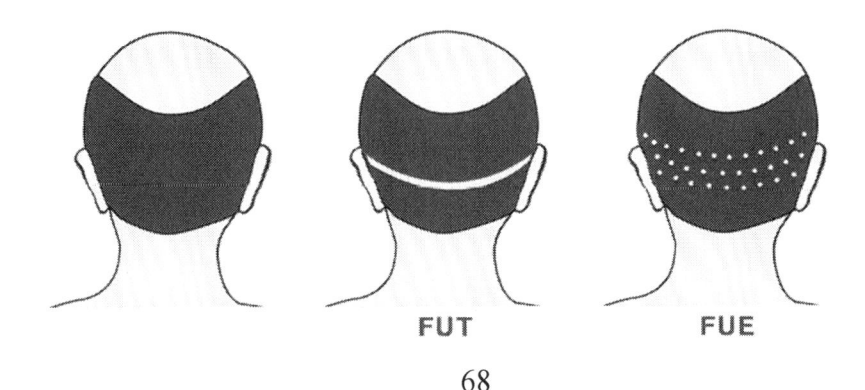

FUT   FUE

Follicular Unit Transplantation (FUT) - Strip Excision Harvesting

This is a common technique whereby a single, double, or triple blade surgical knife is used to harvest the donor tissue bearing the hair strands to be transplanted. Care is taken to ensure that the hair follicles are intact when the tissue is harvested. Once cut out, the hair strip is separated into individual follicles with a cluster of hairs in each. This form of hair extraction results in a linear scar that is covered with time as the hair grows in length.

Follicular Unit Extraction (FUE)

This is the other from of hair extraction where, instead of strips of follicular tissue, individual follicular grafts are harvested. In this case, once the graft is harvested, there is no need to separate the tissue as each graft is harvested in a single unit. Each follicle is made up of 1–4 hair strands, oil glands, muscles, and connecting tissue which are then transplanted as a unit.

This technique results in smaller scars that can easily be covered with the surrounding hair once it grows. Since the follicular grafts are harvested one unit at a time, the procedure takes a lot of time and the cost of each graft is often higher than those produced using strip excision. For these reasons, the procedure using this form of hair harvesting is more expensive, but the end results are much better.

When harvesting donor hair, the strip or incision made when harvesting the hair is determined by the patient's hair density and scalp elasticity. Patients with high density hair require fewer grafts, so the strips or units harvested are few. The elasticity of one's scalp is also considered as patients with tight scalps will only allow small strips to be harvested while those with loose scalps can withstand the harvesting of wider strips with more follicular units.

The size and number of follicles harvested is determined in relation to the tightness and looseness of the scalp to minimize scarring after the operation. Tight scalps require the harvesting of small strips to ensure minimal scarring while loose scalps can allow the harvesting of more grafts and wider follicular strips because they heal better with minimal scars as compared to tight scalps.

Creating the Recipient Sites and Grafting

The harvested hair grafts are inserted into the hair recipient sites which are prepared by making minute slits. Creating well-suited recipient sites is important to achieving consistently satisfactory results in hair restoration. The process requires sophisticated surgical skill and experience, as well as a keen aesthetic sense.

In constructing hair recipient sites, the main objective is to create neat, clean small incisions ready and waiting to receive the new hair follicle implants. First, the recipient site is anesthetized, and then carefully marked according to the plan of operation. Tiny slits are then made on the transplant site where the new hair follicles will be grafted. The surgeon uses a fine instrument to aid the transplant while also using a wide array of incision instruments-- miniblades, needles, micro-punches, etc.,--to create the recipient site "wounds" or openings.

Doctors have preferences as to what instruments they use to make incisions. Some doctors use 16-18 gauge needles which are very small, while others make use of small scalpels to make tiny slits on the skin before squeezing the implants into the opening.

Typically, the incisions made on the recipient site are 0.5 to 2.0 millimeters apart, depending on the location and the size of the grafts. The grafts or follicle implants are placed as close as possible to the frontal hair line. They are also placed in the central or post-frontal areas to pack the new hair densely.

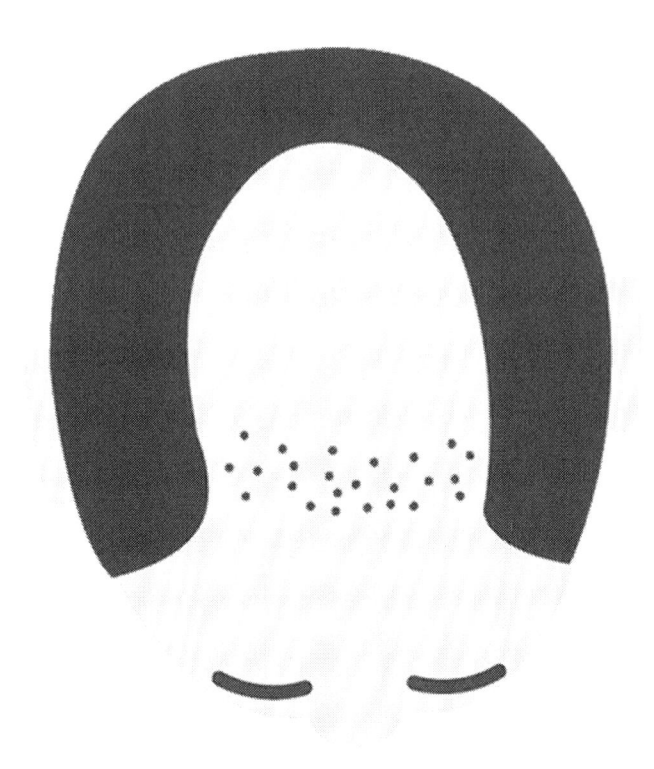

Much of the aesthetic result of the transplant is determined by how the recipient sites were created. The construction of the hair recipient sites sets the angles at which the new hairs will grow, and it determines the density and equal distribution of the hair grafts. Specifically, implant line, density and direction influence the final result of the hair transplant.

Over the years surgeons have used various techniques to perform follicular unit hair transplantation. One such technique is the Lateral Slit Technique. The technique helps give the surgeon the highest control over the angle and direction in which the newly transplanted hair will grow, and ultimately produces superior results.

As soon as the recipient sites are created, the follicular unit micrografts are placed into the slit. One-hair follicular units are used at the frontal hair line to give a natural appearance. The three- and four -graft hair follicles are used in the central forelock location to provide fullness. The placement of the grafts takes time and you are allowed to take a break to use the restroom, if needed; you can also have a snack, stretch, watch TV or sleep.

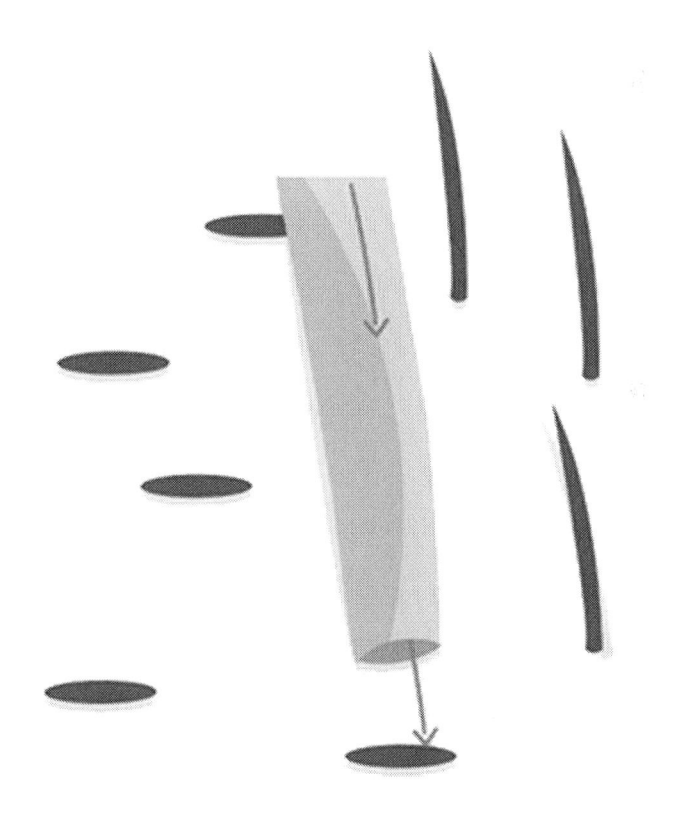

Once the grafts heal and start to receive nutrients, the hair follicles begin to repair themselves and new hair begins to grow.

FUT

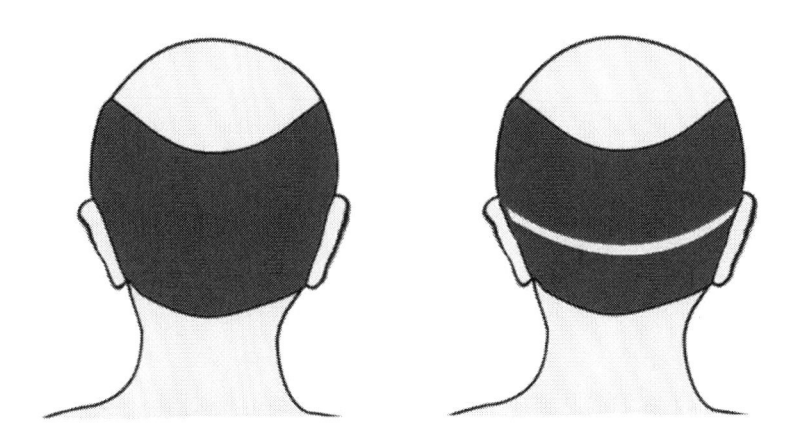

Follicular Unit Transplantation

Follicular Unit Transplantation (FUT)

It has been a challenge for scientists to develop a technique through which hair restoration can be done successfully. After a lot of research and experiments over almost a century, things are looking better with highly advanced technology and in-depth research in this area. One of the latest techniques is Follicular Unit Transplantation, which enables people with baldness to have normal and naturally growing hair again.

What does Follicular Units mean?

With the help of high-resolution microscopes, it was found that hairs do not grow individually. In fact, they grow in tiny groups of 1-4 follicles. These bundles of follicles are called follicular units. Other than follicles, a unit of hair also has 1-2 villus hairs, oil glands, a muscle, nerves, blood vessels, and collagen. It is important to keep this configuration together to make sure that the growth of hair does not get affected.

How a follicular unit transplantation procedure is done

This amazing hi-tech solution for hair restoration came into practice in 1990s. With this highly advanced method, follicle units are extracted safely and grafted into the affected areas of the scalp. It is of utmost importance to keep the hair follicles in the units intact. During its early years in the micro-grafting procedure there were high chances of damaging the hair follicles. But with FUT, it is possible to extract the tissue in one piece without causing any damage through the Single Strip Harvesting technique. Another advanced method, Follicular Unit Extraction (FUE), is also used for safer removal of the intact follicle units.

Other than helping in removal of conserved hair follicles, another benefit of Follicle Unit Transplantation is the use of smaller sites for implant. With the support of powerful microscopes, it is possible to remove non-hair bearing tissues surrounding the small graft size for small hair follicles. Minute needle-sized sites are used to implant the follicular units. The smaller size heals faster and the marks are undetectable.

FUT requires hair to be transplanted in follicular units made up of naturally occurring clumps of 1-4 hair strands. The follicular units are not only made up of the hair strands, but they also come along with small muscles, sebaceous glands, nerves, and other types of tissue that are normally attached to hair follicles. These additional aspects are harvested in one unit, together with the hair strands, and are transplanted as one unit in a single session which increases the chances of the transplanted hair successfully growing after the surgery.

This kind of procedure produces hair growth that follows the same growth pattern as the surrounding hair resulting in a look that is as natural as possible. This is because the follicular units are transplanted one at a time with the surgeon ensuring that they follow the required pattern and are identical to the other follicular units transplanted around it along with the hair that is already growing in the transplant region. The grafts are distributed by the surgeon as evenly as possible so that the overall effect is quite pleasing to the eye and mingles well with surrounding hair growth. This procedure also allows the doctor to make efficient use of the hair grafts harvested.

One thing that makes this procedure a success, as opposed to harvesting hair in a strip, is that in the first place, even before the surgery is done, the surgeon is able to estimate the grafts that are needed for the procedure. Generally, surgeons measure the follicular unit distribution on the scalp at 1 unit per mm. They use this method to measure the transplant region and calculate the number of grafts that will be required for the procedure. They can then harvest just the right amount of grafts needed. In this way, it is easy to plan the details of a hair transplant. This procedure also prevents the harvesting of excess donor hair thereby preserving hair for any future hair transplants should they be needed.

This procedure also results in optimal merging of the harvested hair follicles with the incisions in the transplant region. This minimizes any trauma to the scalp and results in scars that are smaller than those resulting from an FUE transplant. The surgeon trims the excess tissue surrounding the harvested hair grafts by using stereomicroscopic dissection in a way that will prevent any damage to the follicles. The resulting follicle is then just the right size that is required – small, compact, and easily fitted into the tiny incisions made on the transplant region. This minimizes any unnecessary damage to scalp tissue and gives a clean finish with scars that can be easily camouflaged once the hair grows out.

This procedure is also valued because it enables the availability of enough hair follicles to provide a good hairline and also a fuller look since very few hair grafts are wasted. This concludes the information concerning follicular unit transplantation.

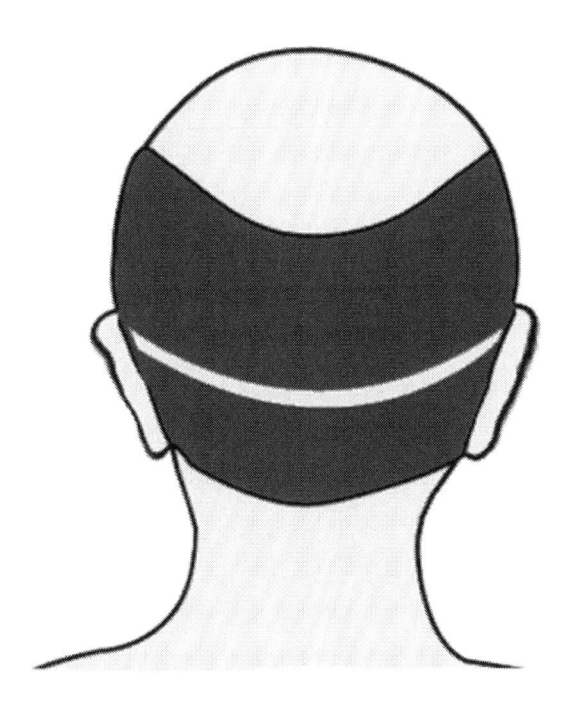

Important Aspects of Follicle Unit Transplantation Surgery

The Follicle Unit Transplantation procedure needs to be planned very carefully, as there are many factors to keep in mind. The most important element in the master plan, prior to starting the surgery, is to remember that the patient might lose hair with time. Hence, the surgery has to be prepared in such a way that the patient never finds himself short of hair in the long term.

Other factors that are involved in the meticulous surgical planning are proper framing of the face, covering the scalp, and sessions.

Proper framing of the face

While preparing for surgery, a suitable frontal hairline needs to be ascertained that will balance with the features of the patient's face. The ideal placement is always the patient's natural hairline. In the event of limited hair from donor, the best option is to keep the implants scarce at the temple and towards the back of the crown areas. The patient's mid-portion of the frontal hairline should not be compromised, as it will affect the appearance. Similarly, creating a higher hairline will not meet the purpose. Instead, it will extend the forehead and misbalance the facial proportions and eventually highlight the baldness.

Covering the scalp

In order to get effective results out of this cosmetic surgery, the first priority should be to fill up the front and top of the bald areas of the scalp in the first session. Only after these areas are filled adequately, should the crown area be taken care of, depending upon the available stock of donor hair. It is easier for the patient to assess the look after the first session of front and top filling. Another session can be done if he desires more density. Once it is done, the areas of crown can be worked upon with the leftover reserve of donor hair.

Large sessions of transplant are beneficial

The cosmetic surgery based on FUT technology lets surgeons perform large sessions of implants on the patients. Large sessions are advantageous. Surgeons are able to give patients a natural look from all angles in the very first session. It also helps in preserving the donor hair, as the number of extractions of hair follicles is reduced. This enables the surgeon to make the best use of the donor hair supply to cover all the planned areas for restoration. The other benefit is that the whole procedure is completed in a short period of time, as longer sessions give faster and more effective results which reduces the time taken in subsequent sessions.

The Procedure of FUT

Before carrying out the transplanting procedure, the surgeon performs a thorough investigation of the medical history of the patient. Among other things, like blood tests, he checks the elasticity of the scalp, as high elasticity means easier extraction of hair follicles.

Change your look with a new hairline

With the FUT procedure, it is possible to get a different hairline. For convenience, the surgeon draws the hairline on the scalp of the patient. If you would want to have a receded hairline so that more of your forehead is visible, you should inform the surgeon. He would draw the new hairline a little farther into the scalp. Similarly, if you would like to have an advanced hairline, the surgeon could cover more area on the scalp and create a new hairline accordingly.

A well-reputed surgeon also has a good sense of aesthetics. Hence, if you are confused regarding the type of hairline that would suit your face, you may discuss it with the surgeon and get good advice.

How does it all begin?

The FUT procedure is carried out by a hair transplant surgeon and a team of assistant surgeons. Right before the transplantation begins, the surgeon goes through a checklist. At this point, they may also confirm a few aspects of the surgery with the patient. Feel free to ask any questions that you may have regarding FUT.

The patient is then asked to assume a reclining position. To keep the patient in a relaxed state, many hair transplantation clinics play relaxing music or offer TV viewing. You could also request to be sedated if you are feeling too anxious.

Administration of Local anesthesia

The FUT procedure begins by giving local anesthesia to the patient. You will be asked to lie down on an operating table and then oral sedatives will be provided for you. It is followed by a dose of the anesthetic shots called either Lidocaine or Xylocaine. This local anesthetic is combined with another longer lasting one known as Bupivicaine or Marcaine.

Local anesthesia's function is to make the scalp area, from where the strip will be collected, numb. It ensures that the sessions are totally painless and devoid of any anxiety for the patient.

Vibratory anesthesia is used to make the administration process comfortable. This method involves using vibration of an elevated frequency on the skin surface. It ensures that when the anesthetics are administered, the patient does not have to go through the uneasiness of sensations that the injections normally engender. Moreover, the needle used to inject anesthetic is very fine and hurts only a little. The doctor also keeps ice packs handy in order to reduce even that little bit of pain.

The anesthetics used are very strong and thus, only the border of the scalp is used for administering them. This part is called a ring block. The interior of the scalp is not touched at all. The whole scalp becomes numb as a result. The time required for performing the entire FUT differs from one case to another. Hence, it is normal for a patient to require further anesthesia shots in a single session.

A surgeon does not wait for the anesthesia to lose its effect and administers a fresh dose before the current one wears off. The surgeon does not let the patient feel any discomfort that could be caused by the surgery procedure. The repetition of the anesthetics is generally sought after a lapse of 5-6 hours.

There are many blood vessels in the scalp area, which is why it is common that any procedure around this part of the body will involve a lot of bleeding. However, this does not happen during FUT surgery.

Advanced technology has made sure that the procedure is accomplished with the least amount of bleeding. Another nice aspect is that the patient is not required to take a lot of medicine. The surgery is carried out with a patient-centric approach. Hence, the procedure has been hailed as a very effective and inviting one for people with a hair loss problem.

Extraction of donor tissue

In FUT, the donor tissue or the hair-bearing skin is extracted from the donor's site and is implanted on the areas of the scalp affected with baldness. The extraction of donor tissue is done as a single strip harvesting process. First, an ideal donor area on the scalp with dense hair is identified, which in most cases, is the back of scalp. It is safer to remove strips of hair-bearing skin from these dense areas, as the surrounding hair will be able to camouflage the affected area well. A tight scalp can make it a little more time-consuming to harvest the strips. The laxity of scalp is important to achieve a smooth and efficient extraction of the follicular unit strips.

Once the donor area is selected, the surgeon harvests thin strips of tissue carefully because the natural configuration of hair follicles need to be kept intact. Extra care is required to keep these extracted crops of hair follicles or follicular units (FUs) alive, as they do not have the natural support of body fluids to survive. Hence, they are immediately placed into a solution, which has same qualities as that of body fluids. The solution keeps the FUs healthy until they are implanted back into the scalp's bald areas.

This technique is useful in removing a large number of hair follicles with minimal damage to the grafts while leaving a thin linear scar on the scalp. These thin scarred wounds are generally closed with the help of self-absorbent sutures or staples and do not take much time to heal. Nevertheless, these scars, when healed, are visible if the patient wears their hair too short or when the hair is wet or when the density of hair around the scar is too thin. To tackle this problem, the trichophytic technique is used. This technique enables the hair to grow through the scar and effectively helps the scar by masking it. Generally, the process of single strip harvesting takes around 15-20 minutes.

Dissection using stereomicroscope

The FUs are generally made of 1-4 hairs each. In FUT, the groups of these FUs on the extracted single strip are required to be separated very carefully. The natural state of these follicular units (FUs) should remain intact when they are being implanted on the scalp, otherwise there will not be healthy hair growth. This process of separating these follicles from the strip is done under the direct vision of a high-end, powerful stereo-microscopic view. The extra tissue and skin are thoroughly dissected and disposed. These FUs are then stored safely after they are sorted according to the number of hair each unit contains.

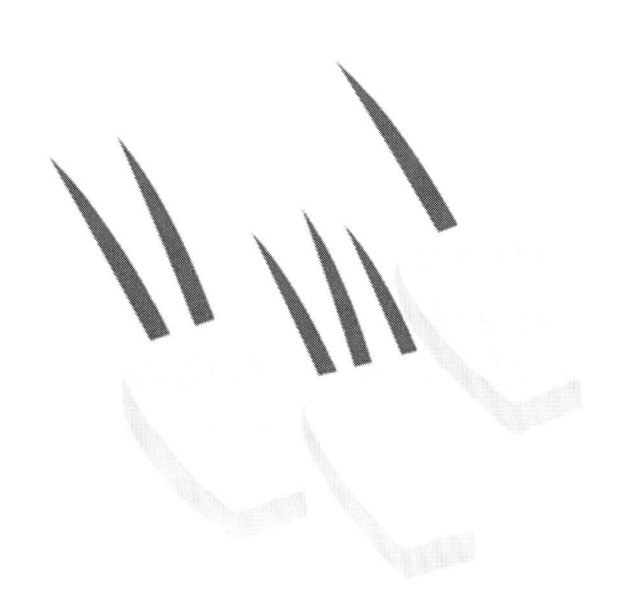

Preparing the recipient area

The recipient area is the portion of the scalp where the transplanted hair follicles are to be placed. The surgeon preps the area by making minute slits. Naturally shaped scores are preferred because they ensure hair growth that would look just like the real hair. The incisions are never too big; they are close to the size of skin pores. It promises very minimum bleeding.

The number of slits that need to be made and other aspects related to them are decided by the surgeon after due consideration. Expert hair transplantation surgeons prepare the recipient area in such a way that the look and density of the new hair is just what the patient would want to have.

Moreover, an experienced surgeon always protects the existence of prevailing natural hair. Surgeons try to do minimum damage to it. Thus, the recipient area is prepared without any cutting or shaving of the actual hair. It allows the patient to cover the recipient area with natural hair until new hair growth takes place.

Placement of FUs

After the recipient site is all prepped, the surgeon and his team would proceed to place the FUs at their designated points. This step is very critical in the FUT procedure. You will be asked to stay as still as possible so that the FUs could be placed perfectly. Depending upon the space of the area that needs to be covered with FUs, the step can take from a few hours to a whole day.

For an all-natural look, the surgeon has to use the FUs strategically. A graft of 4 to 5 FUs is used in the middle of the scalp while single FUs are used to create the hairline. This trick works very well and allows the patient to enjoy the feel of natural hair that grows from the transplanted hair follicles.

As keeping the head in the same position can be a tough task for the patient, you could ask your surgeon for a break whenever you feel like you need one. Do not worry; the long duration of the step will never be an issue for you. To keep the patient busy, most transplantation centers offer magazines, TV viewing, etc. You could also fall asleep. Simply inform the surgeon so that the team could place your head in a comfortable position and you could catch a wink effortlessly. As your scalp will be under the influence of anesthesia, you need not worry about discomfort or pain.

When the surgery is over

After the surgeon and his team have successfully transplanted all the FUs, they will check the recipient's area to ensure that the work has been done to perfection. Then, the head is covered with a bandage resembling a headband. Per your preference, you could wear a cap or a bandana to cover your head from exposure.

Since you were sedated prior to the surgery, you should not drive home. If you have come alone for the surgery, ask your surgeon how long it will be before you are physically fit to drive a vehicle. You could also ask him questions related to the surgery and post-operative care at home. If you are feeling any discomfort, let the surgeon know. Many patients experience pain and swelling in the scalp region and thus, they are given painkillers.

Tips for post-FUT care

- When lying down for a nap or a night's sleep, make sure that your head is placed in a raised position. The height

of 2-3 pillows is perfect for the immediate post-op days. It helps in faster healing of the donor area.
- The bandage is to be removed before you take a shower the following day. Make sure the water is neither too hot nor too cold. Moderately warm water is perfect for your scalp. Do not use strong sprays or stand right under a strong shower, as it could damage the stitches.
- Use a neutral shampoo or the one as recommended by your surgeon for gently washing your head and softly patting the hair dry. Do not worry; shampooing will not cause the transplants to come off.
- Since the stitches are still fresh, you should avoid jerking your head. Any kind of shock to it could cause the stitches to open. Moreover, you should choose to wear upper garments that you can wear without pulling them over your head. It would allow your head to have least interaction with foreign material and facilitate quick healing.
- As for your diet, you can eat regular food items without inhibition. However, you should refrain from consuming alcohol for at least 3 days after surgery. Those who smoke should skip their habit for at least 2 weeks.
- Keep your exercise routine light for a couple of weeks, as heavy perspiration and raised body temperatures could cause delay in healing of the stitches.
- You can revert to normal hair care 10 days after the surgery, as within this duration, the FUs are still getting

properly lodged in the scalp. After the 10th day, you can get a haircut and even get your hair colored.

FUE

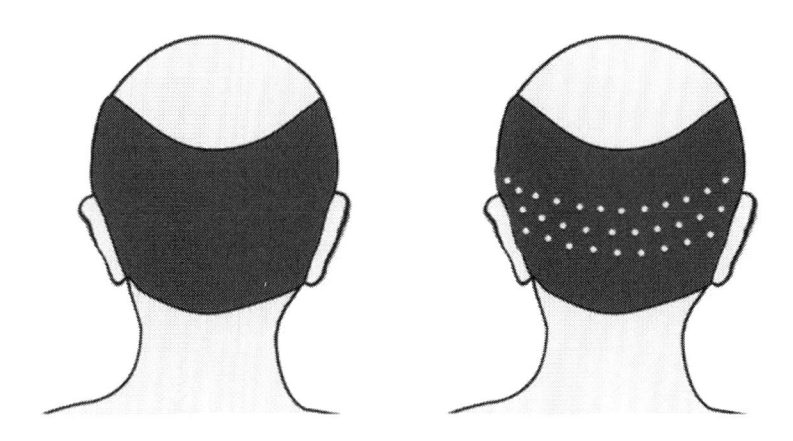

Follicular Unit Extraction

Follicular Unit Extraction (FUE)

Follicular unit extraction (FUE) procedure involves the harvesting of donor hair in individual follicular units. This method was first performed by a Japanese doctor Masumi Inaba, who used to extract hair using a 1 mm. needle. Since then, the procedure has undergone great improvement. However, it requires a lot of skill, and as a result, few have mastered it. There are special follicular extraction tools now in use that were not available in the past, which have made it a faster and more accurate operation.

However, the removal of hair follicle units in their natural state is a very challenging method to perform. . If not done carefully, there are higher chances of damage to the hair follicles' natural components, which are very essential for a proper growth post graft. Hence, the process of FUE takes a long time to complete. Since the area of dermis to which the follicular units are attached is a tight zone, extra care has to be taken by first loosening the zone before pulling out the intact follicle units. Small micro punches sized from 0.6-0.8 mm are used, as the follicular units are very narrow at the surface.

Since the tightness of the zone around dermis varies in patients, it is necessary to do a test first to evaluate if FUE can be performed on the patient. The test is done by pulling out around 100 follicular units and then checking how many of them are in an intact position. If the extraction is easy and most are complete units, only then FUE should be done.

The scarring associated with this form of hair harvesting is referred to as pit scarring. These are small whitish round scars that appear in the donor region where the grafts are harvested. Many people prefer to have pit scarring, as opposed to the linear scarring, resulting from the other form of hair extraction known as follicular unit transplantation.

Follicular unit extraction results in a quicker recovery time after a transplant, as opposed to follicular unit transplantation. There is less discomfort during healing, as well. However, the region from which follicular unit extraction is done is quite wide because it must be done unit by unit. This means that the donor region may exhibit some thinning as a result of the harvesting of the grafts. This is quite possible in people with low hair density. Such an occurrence may make the resulting scars visible which is a disadvantage as most people desire any scars from hair transplant surgery to be hidden under hair growth.

The resulting fragility of the scalp after the hair grafts are harvested means that subsequent harvest sessions will be limited. This is because the scalp region in the donor area has been weakened as it was exposed to trauma when the individual hair grafts are being harvested. The procedure is also more expensive as it requires more time and effort on the part of the technician and doctor doing the hair transplant to get the grafts and transplant them.

It is important to get an in-depth consultation before you settle for this form of hair extraction. Just because it produces better results after the transplant than the other form of extraction, doesn't mean it will be ideal for you. The doctor has to consider the quality of your scalp, the characteristics of your hair, and the extent of your hair loss to choose the right treatment for you.

The skill of the doctor and technicians performing your procedure will also determine the results of the hair harvesting. You should also keep in mind the kind of equipment they use and their facilities as all these will contribute to the overall success of the process.

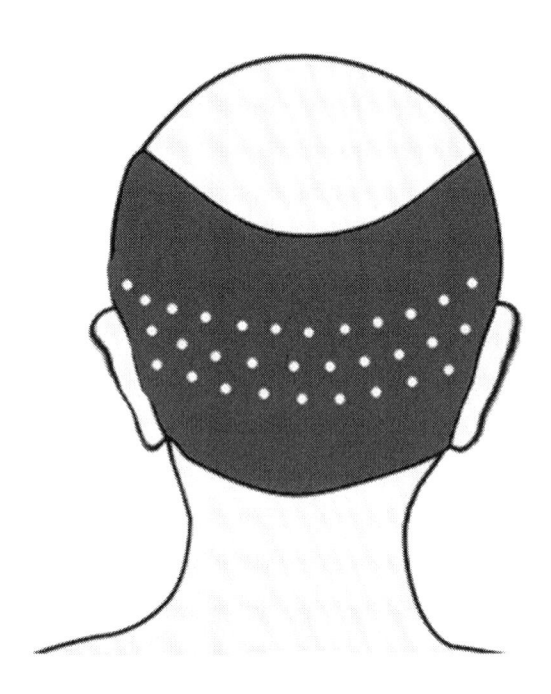

FOX Test: Benchmark for Evaluating Candidacy for FUE

Follicular Unit Extraction has made hair transplantation a very convenient and aesthetically appealing process for the patient. The time taken for recovery after the procedure is very short and the patient can easily sport short hair subsequently. The scars left from the surgery are undetectable. Nevertheless, since this method is based on a successful extraction of intact follicular units from the scalp, the candidacy of the patient has to be determined first for a promising yield in the future.

What is the relevance of FOX test in FUE?

In FUE, the follicular units require direct extraction from the dermis. The strength with which the units hold on to the scalp varies from person to person. If the units are very well ingrained into the scalp, the surgeon may not find it easy to extract the follicular units in their complete form. This is fundamental for the success of this hair restoration technology. Therefore, before the surgeon can go ahead with FUE, he needs to be sure that the patient's scalp is right for conducting this procedure. The FOX test helps decide the candidacy of the person interested in receiving hair restoration through FUE.

What happens during FOX test?

In this test, the doctor examines whether the follicular units from the donor site will still be eligible for implanting fruitfully after extraction. For this purpose, he pulls out around 100 grafts from the scalp. Then, he evaluates the level of ease he experienced during extraction and the status of the units. If the result shows that the units are healthy after extraction and the process was easy, the patient is declared a strong candidate for FUE. The health of the extracted follicular unit is ascertained by biopsy.

Five grades in the FOX test

This test has been categorized into 5 grades that are in accordance with the effortlessness in extraction and intactness of the pulled out grafts.

- The result is categorized in grade 1 when complete follicular units actually come out with the utmost ease or if only rare transection of each hair is found in the unit.
- It is grade 2 when the act of extraction does not require much effort in the initial session. However, as the donor site starts becoming scarred, the following sessions present a lot of difficulty, and the extracted units are not available in the desired form. Hence, the long-term hair growth may not be very promising.
- Grade 3 result happens with the patients with which the emergent angle is not easy.
- In grades 4 and 5, the surgeon is not able to envisage the emergent angle with certainty. It is definite that hair growth, if the surgery is done on patients of these grades, will be very poor. The chance of elevated transection rate is nearly always confirmed in these cases.

Grade 1-3 patients are declared good candidates for FUE while those with grades 4-5 are advised of other techniques for hair restoration. The results of the FOX test may not prove constant if done on the same patient again after some time. The variation occurs because of repeated access of the same donor site for extraction.

Surgical Procedure of FUE

The surgical process of FUE needs a lot of meticulous preparations, expert knowledge, and skill to perform it. Hence, it is a slow process. However, the great results achieved after FUE hair transplantation beautifully compensate for the time spent.

The surgical process starts with trimming the hair on the back of the head, identified as the donor site, to 1-2 mm in length. The patient lies in a prone position and the donor site on the scalp is then anesthetized slowly.

The follicular units are narrow on the surface; hence, micro-punches with small diameters between 0.6 and 1 mm are used to harvest them carefully in several steps as follows:

- The protective skin around the follicular unit to be removed is marked with the sharp side of the micro-punch.
- The hair unit is then loosened by twisting it with the blunt side of the punch while pushing it deeper under the skin.
- Finally, the follicular unit is slowly pulled out in its natural state with the help of forceps. In order to preserve them, they are stored in a solution, which is identical to body fluids.
- After the required amount of extraction is done, the follicular units are implanted on the affected area of the scalp.

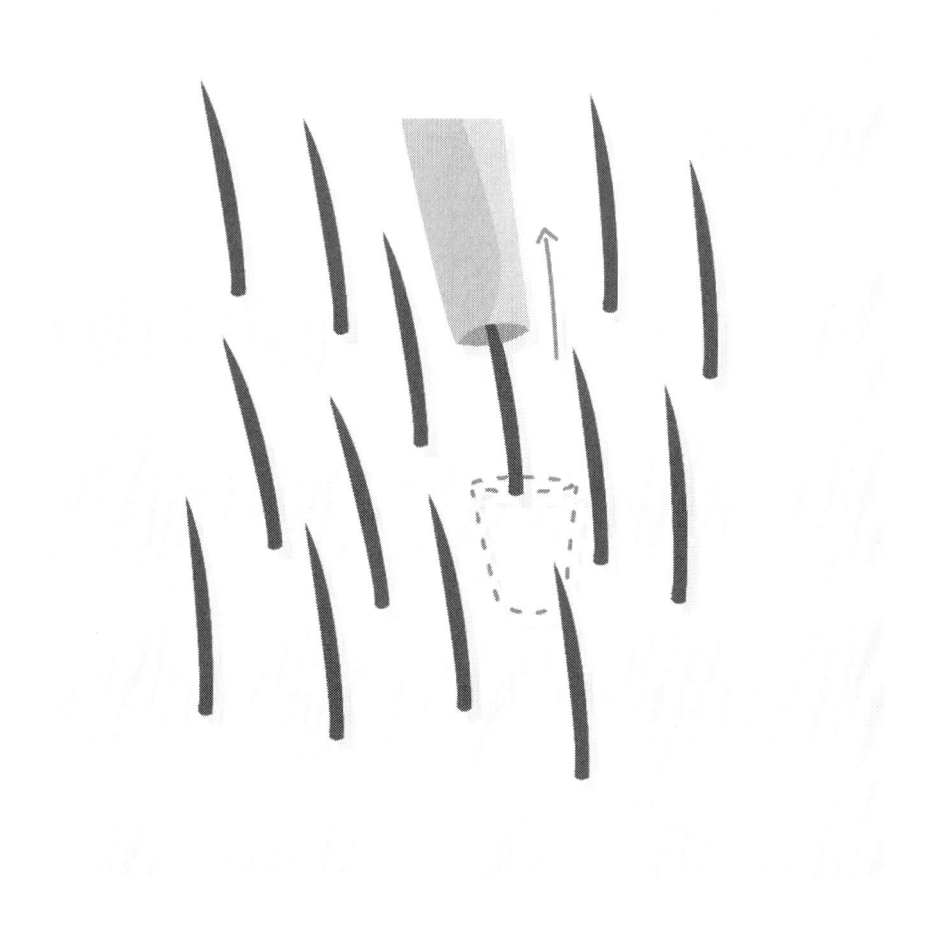

Extraction in FUE is performed in order to harvest hair follicles from the patient's head or other area(s) of the body with the aim of transplanting them on the bald area. Hair transplant surgeons follow either of the following two steps for extraction:

Two-step procedure

After placing a sharp punch over the follicular unit, keeping in mind the direction of the hair, the second step is to pull out the follicle slowly by gripping the top of the follicular unit. The punch should not be pushed deeper to protect the root from possible damage.

- **First step**

A punch measuring 1 mm is used to surround a follicular unit (FU). Its placement is important, as most transections (hair follicle damage) occur due to its incorrect placement. The surgeon has to make sure that the punch follows the direction of hair shaft. Next, with a circular movement of the punch, the surgeon penetrates the upper layer of the scalp and succeeds in separating the FU from its surrounding tissues.

- **Second step**

The surgeon now uses special surgical forceps to give the head of the FU a gentle twist, which causes it to become loose. He then pulls it away. In case the FU does not become loose, then the surgeon is required to perform another step. He goes deeper into the skin and tracts the FU using a U-shaped dissection needle.

Three-step procedure

The abovementioned 2-step procedure causes a number of transections, which makes the extraction process time consuming for the patient and tiring for the surgeon. Dr. James Harris of the

International Society of Hair Restoration Surgery succeeded in lowering the percentage of transections by performing one more step in the FU extraction. He added an additional third step with new instrumentation. With a blunt instrument he was able to minimize damage to follicles during the process of separating the follicular unit from the surrounding donor tissue.

First, a sharp punch is used to score the protective outer layer of the skin (i.e. epidermis). Then, a blunt punch is applied to the area and with a minor tugging and to and fro movement, the FU is dislodged from the skin. Lastly, surgical forceps are used to pull out the FU in its intact form. He found that the graft yield increased from 92% by two-step technique to 98%; and the hair yield improved from 74 to 93% by using the three-step technique.

Are there any disadvantages of the 3-step procedure?

The three-step procedure, however, fails to deal with buried grafts. During the FUE extraction, often times the hair grafts are unintentionally pushed deeper into the skin, which result in buried grafts. A surgeon could leave such grafts as they are. Nevertheless, in many patients, they cause cysts. Hence, it becomes mandatory for the doctor to remove buried grafts during the FUE procedure.

If the grafts are not buried deep enough, they can be pulled out using an instrument called the Shamberg extractor. In case they are too deep, a surgical scalpel is used to pull them out.

Can buried grafts be avoided?

Surgeons can avoid buried grafts by following these suggestions:

- Refrain from choosing the back of the head as the donor area. There, the hair grows out in an acute angle, which risks buried grafts.
- Shift the angle of the instruments for the location of the FUs.
- Trim the hair at the donor area as much as possible.
- If the patient has coarse hair, the 2-step procedure may be a better option.

Pros and Cons of FUE in Hair Grafting

Follicular Unit Extraction is the latest method in hair transplantation. Like any other technologically advanced methods, this one also has its own issues and benefits.

Advantages

- The traditional single strip graft method leaves a long scar on the donor site of the scalp. This becomes a cosmetic issue for patients desiring to wear shorter hair. Even with the trichophytic technique, the visibility of these linear scars do not disappear completely. Hence, for people who want to wear their hair short whenever they wish after the graft, FUE is a better alternative. It leaves very small dot-like scars, which are almost undetectable, even with shorter hair.
- After the procedure, the patient is allowed to do exhaustive physical workouts.

- It is the best option for the people who are suffering from partial hair loss like androgenic alopecia or small balding areas on top. It is an ideal procedure for other cosmetic issues like widow's peak (i.e. loss of hair on forehead in triangular area in women), moustaches, eyebrows, eyelashes etc.

- Many patients opting for hair transplant do not have the required scalp laxity because their skin is too tight for single strip method. In this case, FUE is a better option for them to restore hair growth.
- FUE is very useful in cases where there are scars from earlier strip procedures allowing no additional single strip methods.
- Linear scars from strip method take a long time to heal in some patients. Hence, the FUE procedure is a better choice, as the scars are very small and take less time to heal.
- This procedure is advantageous for patients suffering from excessive fear of pain and scarring because the incision is less painful and the resultant scars are negligible.
- There is no need to visit the surgeon for stitch removal from the healed wounds.
- This method is very useful even to cover the earlier linear scars from strip harvesting.

- This is the only technique which enables the surgeon to use body hair to also give required density to the hair transplant.

Disadvantages

- Since FUE is a slow and tiresome procedure, it takes a lot of patience and energy in a surgeon. He requires taking short breaks, as the prolonged posture affects his neck muscles.
- Highly skilled hands are required to perform this procedure. In-depth knowledge and experience is necessary to know the connection between the exit and under-the-skin angle of the follicle. Lack of knowledge can render a higher rate of transection to the follicles. Higher rate of damage would risk the supply of enough hair follicle units needed for grafting onto the affected bald area.
- The long duration of this process causes a lot of uneasiness to the patient because of continuously being in the same (prone) position.
- Due to the time-consuming factor, the follicular extractions are limited. Hence, it takes multiple sessions over several days to yield the required follicles for grafting.
- The method is expensive, as it takes quite a long time to complete.

Though this procedure has been accepted well by both doctors and patients, research is going on to find ways to cut short the duration and minimize the transection rate of the follicles, which would eventually help in bringing down the cost of the FUE procedure.

Innovations in FUE

Although FUE is an advanced procedure in itself, the scope for improvement is always there. The focus of bringing in innovation to this technique is to make it as comfortable for the patient as possible. Hair transplant surgeons and companies dedicated to providing advanced hair transplant equipment are researching tirelessly for innovations in FUE.

What challenges does traditional FUE hold?

The foremost challenge that a surgeon faces while performing this surgery is the selection of hair follicles in the donor area. It is true that the rear side of the scalp is an ideal donor area, but the quality of hair follicles also matters. Since it is impossible to see inside the scalp and determine the healthiness of a follicle, a surgeon has to choose them randomly.

Second, while extracting hair follicles manually, transection (breaking up of follicles) occurs. Even a highly experienced hair transplant surgeon has a transection rate of 5%.

Third, in order to leave the minimum post-extraction impact on the donor area, a surgeon has to be extremely precise while performing follicle extraction. Using a surgical tool, they need to make an incision around a hair follicle and delicately pull it from its place. They carry on with this process until they have pulled enough follicles to cover the recipient area.

Of course, hair follicle extraction performed in this way is time consuming and the surgeon is hard pressed to work with precision. A little extra incision into the scalp surface could mean a deeper scar and extra healing time for the patient.

Due to the above mentioned imperfections, many surgeons have now embraced a new technology in FUE, which is as follows:

Use of equipment in FUE

SAFE System is a device that excels in successful separation of the hair follicle from its surrounding skin. It is a handheld device and makes rotational movements to enter the scalp softly. Another device that works the same way is called Rotocore. This equipment is also handheld, but saves more time by helping the surgeon make a straight incision. It removes any chances of transection.

Moreover, the device prevents any deeper incision than required for extraction. Before, the surgeon was required to measure the incision depth needed to extract the hair follicle intact. Now, they select the depth measurement on the panel on the device and let the device make a smooth removal.

Complete automation in FUE

The robotic system makes FUE a seamless procedure for the surgeon and experience has fewer scars for the patient. The system is fully equipped to perform every step of the FUE with complete perfection. It begins the procedure by identifying the healthiest hair follicles for extraction. It scans the patient's scalp and analyzes every hair, and removes the need for manual extraction of hair follicles.

The hair follicles are extracted in such a way that the donor area does not have any visible scars. A patient with hair transplantation done via a robotic system can wear his hair short. Neo graft is another automated system wherein the follicles are extracted using pneumatic pressure. It eases hair follicle removal and also facilitates the immediate re-positioning of the follicles. Overall, the surgery time is considerably reduced.

Comparisons between FUT and FUE

Achieving a look of naturally growing hair is the most important aspect of the hair transplantation procedure. The creation of a natural hairline and a good density of hair are equally important for a realistic result. Such close-to-natural looks can be achieved only with the use of in-depth research results and advancements in hair transplantation that have taken place over the last several decades.

Importance of extraction in transplants

The most crucial factor of hair transplantation is the process by which the hair follicular units are harvested. The quality of the harvested follicular units is more important than the quantity of the same. If more of the harvested follicles are damaged due to lack of efficiency or the process itself, then a successful transplant cannot be performed. In FUT, a single strip method is applied by which a strip of hair-bearing skin is removed from the back of the scalp. Then the follicular units are dissected for grafting. In FUE, the process is more developed and specific. Small punch needles are used to carefully to pull out the follicles directly from the donor site of the scalp.

The scars from FUT and FUE

There is a wide difference between FUT and FUE when it comes to the resultant scars from the harvesting. While the strip method in FUT leaves a thin scar running from side to side, the small sized punches in FUE leave only dot-like small scars after the removal of the follicles from the donor area. Although, there is an option to minimize the visibility of the linear scars from FUT through the trichophytic closure method, these scars can still be detected if the hair is worn short. These scars also take a long time to heal. However, with FUE, the dot-like tiny scars are almost invisible even in short hairstyles and take less time to heal.

The sensitivity of follicular units in FUT and FUE

The harvested follicular units through both methods are equally exposed to dehydration. Hence, extra care is required in keeping them healthy before being implanted on the affected areas. These extracted follicular units are stored carefully in a chemical, which have same qualities as that of natural fluids that normally keep them alive.

In the process of extraction, the possibilities of damage to the hair follicles while harvesting is almost same in both FUT and FUE. However, the follicles extracted in FUE are more vulnerable since there is not a lot of protective tissue left around them; this affects their chances of survival.

Implantation of follicular units in FUT and FUE

Although, there is a difference in the way the follicles are extracted in FUT and FUE, the implanting process is same. The skill, experience, and knowledge of the surgeon and his team are the deciding factors in the success of the transplantation process. It has to be done aesthetically for which the surgeon chooses the right number of implants required on the recipient site to achieve a proper density for a balanced look.

The hairline creation is another important factor while implanting, which should match the facial features of the patient. The incision on the recipient's site for implants is a crucial step. The direction, depth, and angle of these incisions should match with the natural hair of the patient. It also helps the roots to connect to the blood vessels and nerves, which ups their survival rate plus the implant looks very natural.

	FUT	**FUE**
Donor area	Back and sides of head	Head and other body parts
Donor area pain after surgery	Moderate	Minimal
Surgical Operating Time/2000 grafts	Less (5-8 hours)	Almost double the FUT (10-12 hours)
Scars in donor area	Linear scar	No visible scars
Healing time of donor area	10-14 Days	3-4 Days
Risk of bleeding & nerve damage	Low	Very low
Cost	Lower	Higher

Robotic Hair Transplant
The Latest Technique with High-Accuracy Results

Many changes have taken place in the field of hair transplantation over the decades. The follicular unit extraction method has made it possible for surgeons to remove donor hair without leaving any noticeable scars on the scalp. The process has become more advanced now with robotic support.

Outline of robotic hair transplant

With the help of this highly advanced technology, the FUE procedure has become more refined and faster. Earlier in FUE procedure, the chances of damage to follicles were higher. Hence, the process was performed very slowly and needed multiple sessions to extract the required number of hair follicles for grafting onto the affected areas.

The ARTAS® Robotic System became popular in 2002 and has now become an integral part of FUE. It is also called R-FUE (Robotic-Follicular Unit Extraction). Besides assisting in the removal of hair follicles, it helps in creating recipient areas using computerized imaging.

Benefits of robotic hair transplant

The most prominent benefits of robot-assisted extraction of hair follicular units are:

- Level of accuracy is very high in locating and removing the follicles safely with less chance of damaging them.

- The time taken in extracting the follicles has been reduced considerably.
- The survival rate of the follicles is higher.
- It can be performed on diversified patients.

Through the FUE method, the follicular units are pulled out directly from the donor areas of the scalp. Each unit consists of 1-4 hairs. The process of extraction is done in two steps.

- The follicular units are separated from the dermis.
- The extracted follicular units are then separated from the attached tissue.

This method and the requirement of separating the follicular units from the protective skin demands a high level of accuracy in order to protect them from any damage. Since this step was done manually for hundreds to thousands of times, it became tedious and laborious. The punch had to be placed exactly at the center of the follicular unit and the dissection had to be done meticulously according to the alignment of the hair with the blunt part of the punch. This task has been a major challenge for surgeons to avoid damage to the natural state of the hair units.

The robot-aided system has resolved this issue to a great extent, as it is possible to separate the follicular units more accurately now. It is a very adaptable technique which can be used for extracting follicles in patients with different racial backgrounds. It also enables the removal of follicles from the sides of the scalp, which was difficult to do manually.

The robotic system process

This highly advanced and innovative technique, which is image-guided, has a robotic arm and dual-needle punch system. The complex method of extraction is done with imaging support. The double-needled punch works with outstanding precision. Its sharp part cuts through the protective skin and the outer blunt part dissects the follicular units from the attached tissue carefully enough to keep them from being injured.

Although the robotic system is hassle-free and gives an excellent outcome while requiring less human participation, the results are still dependent on the doctor's level of experience and efficiency.

With outstanding harvesting results, the robotic system of transplants has become a persuasive process for numerous patients.

How Racial Variation Affects Hair Transplantation

Racial characteristics make a Caucasian individual look different from an African or an Asian. Apart from the color of the skin, the type of hair and its looks differ too. These interesting differences could pose challenges for the surgeon. However, by studying the characteristics and keeping an open mind, hair transplantation can be done perfectly for all races.

Asian hair transplantation

Asian hair is generally black in shade, coarse to the touch, straight, and low in density. The hair, as it grows, sticks away from the root. Coarse hair offers a big advantage for hair transplantation, as its diameter is wider than other kinds of hair. Hence, coarse hair provides more volume and helps cover the recipient area without much effort.

However, since the hairline consists of soft hair, a surgeon may face problems while transplanting the coarse hair on the hairline. The best way to deal with it is to cut off the lower portion of the hair follicle. It provides a soft textured hair that can give an exceptionally good looking natural hairline.

The Asian scalp has a fair complexion, which contrasts greatly with the dark shade of the hair. Moreover, the hair has the tendency of standing out rather than lying flat close to the scalp. Hence, for covering the bald area and lending it a fuller look, the surgeon is required to supply the area with more follicular units (FUs) than generally required for covering a Caucasian head.

African hair transplantation

African hair is thick and mostly curly. The curliness allows for better coverage, as every curl covers more area than straight hair. Unlike Asian scalp, there is little or no color contrast between the scalp and hair. Undoubtedly, Africans or African Americans are good candidates for hair transplantation.

Nevertheless, one challenge that this type of hair presents is its rigidness. While curls can give the feel of fullness, bald areas run the risk of revealing themselves if the patient wears his/her hair loose. The hair cannot be combed in a certain way and be made to cover the bald areas. For this reason, the hair transplant surgeon is required to cover every patch of bald area with hair.

Hair extraction of an individual of African descent needs a different approach, as the type of hair varies. Hair that has soft curls is generally straight under the scalp and thus can be extracted very easily. On the other hand, tightly curled hair has a curly base making the follicle a little larger than the other type. That is why the surgeon has to make a bigger incision in order to extract the hair follicle in its natural state. Similarly, for transplanting such a large-sized hair follicle, enough space has to be created in the recipient's bald area as well.

Planning for Future Hair Loss

Now that you know about the different procedures used in hair restoration surgery, how it's done and how to finance it among other essential factors surrounding it, you need to consider that the hair transplant may be rendered void should you experience future hair loss. So how do you prepare for future hair loss after a hair transplant surgery?

The loss of hair after a hair transplant is referred to as hair transplant shock loss or telogen effluvium. This problem can occur in a number of ways. The first way that this problem can occur is if the hair is transplanted between or around already existing hair. The surgery can cause the underlying hair to fall out due to trauma caused by the surgery. This can happen a few days after surgery, or months after. The only way that this can be avoided is if the already existing hair is stabilized to stay on the head for a long time to come based on the stage it is at on the hair-growth cycle. Then the transplanted hair will have a chance to settle and grow and this will result in harmonious hair growth and a successful hair transplant.

The second way that shock hair loss can occur after a transplant normally occurs after a second hair transplant procedure. This kind of surgery is done to increase the density of hair in an area by some individuals. Unfortunately in some cases the hair that was transplanted in the first procedure falls out or shocks out. However, in this case the hair will grow back. It is just a side effect of the hair transplant, but the hair follicles will recover after some time and produce a new growth of hair.

This kind of shock loss frequently happens with women. The good news is that the hair will grow back. The only thing is that it will take some time, in some cases up to a year, for this to happen. In such cases, patients are advised to apply topical treatments such as Minoxidil to encourage the new hair growth.

Shedding of transplanted hair is the other way in which hair falls off after a transplant procedure. This normally occurs 2-4 weeks after the restoration procedure whereby most, if not all, of the transplanted hair is lost. There is no need to panic as the hair roots and grafts are normally healthy, which means that new hair will gradually grow out of them as the hair transplant settles in. Therefore, you have to wait for some time after shock hair loss to see if the problem will resolve itself.

This normally occurs about 4 months after the operation. The new hair feels like the small stubble that sprouts on skin after a day or two of shaving. These hairs will slowly mature, and after a year, the growth will be quite visible and encouraging, and you can consider the hair transplant surgery a success.

If your hair falls off after a transplant because of progressive balding, then the only thing to do is to see your doctor and prepare for a corrective hair transplant. To avoid such a situation, doctors advise patients to wait for their hair loss to stabilize before they go for a hair transplant.

If after your procedure the doctor warns you of a likelihood of future hair loss, you must do everything to preserve the hair in your donor region. In addition, you need to use medication to minimize the amount of hair loss that will occur after your surgery. Lastly you need to prepare and save the funds you will need for the future surgery.

The good thing is that if you do enough consultation before a procedure and take care to get the right specialists, you will be guided in a way that will keep you from dealing with future hair loss after hair transplant surgery.

Post-Operative Care after Hair Transplant Surgery

Many people agree that finding the correct hair transplant specialist and getting the hair transplant done successfully is a big challenge. After that, one only needs to invest time and self-care to make sure that they heal properly, and everything will turn out fine. However, if you do not take good care of yourself after the surgery, then you may end up ruining work that has taken a lot of time, money and skill to accomplish. So what can you do to ensure a quick and excellent recovery after a hair transplant?

First, follow the doctor's post-operative instructions. Many doctors familiarize hair transplant candidates with these instructions even before they go for the surgery so that they can know them and prepare themselves for the instructions. This ensures that, after the surgery, everything moves along smoothly.

It is common for patients to be given a post-operative pack containing medicine such as mild pain relievers and antibiotics that they need as they recover. Some also give the patient some mild sedatives to help them sleep comfortably for the first few days as the scalp is normally tender and there is a bit of discomfort.

The issue of sleeping arrangements is also a necessary discussion because you need to support yourself in a position that will ensure that you do not disturb the surgery work. Based on where the surgery has been performed it is important to elevate the transplant section on pillows at an angle of 45 degrees. This is another reason for the sleeping tablets given to patients as they require something to induce sleep in this uncomfortable position. This sleeping position is good for preventing swelling, which is a common problem after a hair transplant operation.

After hair transplant surgery, patients are advised to keep the scalp clean at all times. They are advised to start shampooing the scalp on the second day after the surgery as this will help to clear any spots of blood, any scab formations and any oil produced by the hair follicles. Following this, the scalp will be clear of any scabs after seven days. When you make sure the scalp is clean at all times, you prevent any infection from occurring, as infection will hasten the shedding of transplanted hair grafts as they give way to a new growth phase.

In case of itching, which is quite common after surgery, patients are advised to spray the transplant region with saline solution. This will not only reduce the tendency of the region to itch, but it will also promote healing. The post-operative pack given to patients after the surgery in some cases may also include a cream for application on the transplant region to deal with any excessive itching. This depends on the surgeon doing the transplant.

Follow your surgeon's instructions on how to treat the transplant region for the best results. It is also important that you consider temporary measures, such as hats, to put on the region if you are planning to go out in public soon after the surgery. This will help you to avoid unnecessary questions that you may not be ready to answer, and it will help to keep the area covered until the healing process is successful and hair starts to grow in.

It is important that you refrain from heavy activity after the surgery because it will give your scalp time to heal. In fact, many are advised to rest for a fortnight after the surgery before regaining normal activity. In time, you will see if your hair transplant has been successful. You will also find that as your hair loss progresses these areas will be visible after the transplanted hair starts to grow. Once this happens you will be able to decide how to proceed if there are concerns about getting another hair transplant with your doctor. Frequent checkups are required so that the doctor can monitor how the transplanted hair is behaving and for you to know if you need a follow up operation in the future. In addition, the checkups will help you to identify and deal with any complications as they occur.

Possible Side Effects and Complications

Like any other surgery, hair transplants can also result in side effects and complications. Although this procedure is generally considered safe, it is not devoid of risks. Some of these risks are minimized by using a reputable doctor for the transplant. Other side effects occur in spite of a successful procedure and sometimes cannot be avoided. It is good that one familiarizes himself or herself with the complications that can occur during and after hair transplant surgery so that they can better prepare themselves.

The possible side effects and complications differ from person to person. They are as follows:

- **Hemorrhages and infections**

These are common side effects of hair grafting. They can occur during or after the procedure and are normally a result of the doctor not making incisions in the correct way. Infections can occur if the surgery is done in unhygienic surroundings or when unhygienic instruments are used. To avoid this go to an experienced doctor with a fully equipped and state-of-the-art facility. They should also work with experienced technicians who know what they are doing.

- **Transplanted hair falling out**

This normally occurs due to the use of poor technique when carrying out a hair transplant whereby not all hairs transplanted are viable. This means that some of the transplanted hairs will eventually fall out. When you get a good doctor, he/she will have the experience to know when and how to transplant the hair. Your doctor also will have the right technicians who will be able to select viable hair grafts that will be healthy and grow after the transplant.

- **Severe itching**

It is common for some itching to be experienced after a hair transplant, but sometimes it is excessive to the extent of interfering with the healing process and threatening to make the procedure a failure. In such a case, it is important to notify the doctor as he will administer some helpful topical medication to help deal with the issue.

- **Cyst formations**

These occur when the transplanted hair follicles are damaged deep within the skin layer. When this occurs, it is necessary to see the doctor so that corrective measures may be done.

- **Extensive swelling**

It is common for people to experience a bit of swelling as the transplant and donor regions are sensitive after the surgery. However, in some cases it gets out of hand and spreads from the scalp to affect areas like the eyes and forehead. This signifies a severe problem, and while minor swelling on the scalp can be dealt with by using ice packs, a severe case must be given to the surgeon so that he can identify the problem and stop it from occurring.

- **Numbness and pain**

This is a common side effect of the surgery. However, as the days move along and the healing progresses, the numbness and pain dissipate as the transplanted grafts settle in and the anesthesia wears off.

These are some of the side effects you can expect after hair transplant surgery. They can be avoided by taking your time in choosing an expert doctor who works with an expert team of technicians in excellent surroundings, where the necessary equipment and machinery are available. This requires that you choose the hair transplant practice you will use with care and use a doctor with a lot of experience and a good track record.

Caring for Your Hair after Surgery

The way that you care for your hair after surgery really matters when it comes to the healing process. It also determines the results of the hair transplant procedure in the long run.

Normally, when patients leave the practice after the surgery, they are given bottles with sterile solutions that they can apply on the transplanted area and the stitches on the donor area every hour for the first 12 hours after the surgery. This is one reason why it is important to schedule some recovery time after the surgery where you can stay home and attend to your wounds as you cannot do some of these things when you are at work.

Spraying helps to reduce any itching after the surgery and stimulates healing in the area. This keeps one from having to touch the transplant and donor areas as this may spread infection to the region. This spraying also keeps excess scabs from forming and keeps the grafts moist at all times to ensure that they heal well.

You are also advised to wash the region gently with an antiseptic shampoo such as a tea tree oil shampoo to clean out any scabs and blood formed on the donor and transplant regions. Shampooing is not done the regular way. Rather, you should dissolve the shampoo in tepid water and pour or spray the solution all over the scalp, emphasizing the transplanted and donor areas. Rinse after with clean water and pat gently with a towel to dry.

This technique of using a spray bottle for shampooing will continue until two weeks after the transplant. At this stage, you will be expected to visit your doctor for any sutures to be removed. After this, you can revert to your normal shampoo technique and rub the scalp with both hands to dislodge any crusts that remain in the transplant and donor regions. Based on the state of the scalp, the doctor will advise you on when to revert to using products such as gels and hair sprays.

One thing you will be advised to use is medication such as Minoxidil or Rogaine to encourage growth in the transplant region. This is normally prescribed for use until six months after the operation. In the meantime, you will be advised to avoid strenuous activities such as heavy lifting or sports to avoid stretching the transplant region and disturbing the scars.

Expect the transplanted hair to begin to fall out 2–4 weeks after the surgery. You will only notice thin hair growth 3–4 months after the surgery. Six months after the surgery, you will be able to see hair on 70 percent of the transplant region, but fully grown hair will appear at about a year to a year and a half after the surgery. In the case of shock shedding, do not be alarmed as this hair will grow back in time.

Some people choose to take a vacation as they heal from their surgery. If you decide to do so, then avoid sunbathing or using sun lotions on the scalp for the first 2–3 weeks after the surgery. Use a cap on your head if you have to go out in the sun, although it is advisable to keep out of it.

When the Results of a Hair Transplant are Unsatisfactory

Getting an unfavorable result after a hair transplant is not something that many people want to consider, but it does happen to certain individuals. This kind of scenario normally happens either due to an error of judgment on the part of the patient or an error in technique on the side of the specialist.

In case of an error of judgment, it means that the transplant was done too early - at a time when the hair loss was still in progress. In such a case, even if the hair transplant is successful, the hair will still continue to fall out - something that will result in a bald patch forming right after the transplant, resulting in an unnatural look.

The error in technique can occur when the specialist transplants the hair at an abnormal angle such that the new hair growth is facing the wrong way and ends up looking out of place. Other errors include improper donor site closure, poor graft preparation and a poor design of the transplant region resulting in an unattractive look. This is unacceptable as the purpose of a transplant is not only to put hair on a bald spot but to come up with as natural a hairline as possible.

Once you identify the fact that the hair transplant has not achieved the results that you desired, you have the option of getting corrective surgery. Another solution is that you can find other ways of camouflaging the problem, such as using hair pieces.

Getting corrective surgery after a bad hair transplant is a good idea, as opposed to having to deal with the results of a botched hair transplant. However, many people are unable to undergo corrective surgery because they do not have the funds to accomplish this. Instead, they end up where they started -- having to deal with low self-esteem due to bad looking hair.

This is a very difficult position to find yourself in. This is why it is important that everything possible is done to ensure that you get a good quality hair transplant. This means getting the right doctor and making sure that he/she can deliver the kind of results you are looking for based on reviews of past procedures they have done on other people.

If you have funds, then corrective hair surgery is always an option. There are experts that work at correcting bad hair transplants. The main problem with many botched hair transplants is that they do not look natural. A corrective hair surgery can ensure that a bad hair transplant is repaired to look as natural as possible.

If you find that corrective surgery is beyond your reach financially, you have to explore the use of hair systems to help cover the results of the bad hair transplant until you obtain the money to undergo the corrective surgery that is suitable for you. All in all, adequate preparation will prevent you from getting a bad hair transplant in the first place, hence this is the ideal place to focus to keep from getting to a point where you need corrective surgery.

Hair Transplant Repair

While there are a lot of great doctors that do wonderful hair transplants, it is common to find that some patients have fallen victim to bad hair transplants. Dealing with a bad hair transplant especially after suffering from hair loss can be quite traumatizing. Some people don't know how to deal with such a situation and end up living with the results of the botched hair transplant. This is unnecessary as there are professionals that are good at repairing bad hair transplants. The available services for this form of surgery include:

- **Repairing outdated hair transplant procedures**

Outdated hair transplant services are the cause of many negative hair transplants. They normally result in artificial-looking results that feature large hair plugs and excessive scarring. In the case of large hair plugs, corrective surgery can be done and the large hair plugs can be minimized, with the resulting small group of hair strands redistributed to any empty spaces on the scalp.

- **Transplanting hair grafts to hide scarring**

In the case of excessive scarring, the scars can be hidden by transplanting hair grafts directly onto the scar. The other option with scarring is scar revision. This procedure changes the direction that the scar is facing and ensures that it is not visible to an observer. These scars can also be treated using cosmetic solutions such as dermabrasion. With an expert hair surgeon, there is no end to the solutions available for an individual that has negative hair transplant results.

- **Undoing the transplant and starting afresh**

The other hair transplant failure results from the punch graft technique. In this type of hair transplant, the hair at the center of the plug may not grow, which means that the result is a small bald spot at the center of the graft surrounded by hair. This gives a funny look and is the result of the wastage associated with the punch graft technique. To repair such a problem, the doctor can choose to camouflage it using a large number of follicular units that will grow and eventually hide the plugs. The other technique is undoing the grafts and transplanting them one by one as follicular units - in other words repeating the job.

- **Electrolysis and Dermabrasion**

If a small number of hair grafts are placed in the wrong direction and end up facing the wrong way, then there is no need of undoing them and redoing them all again. The unsightly grafts can be destroyed using electrolysis. Healthy hair strands can be transplanted in their place which saves time, as opposed to undoing the unsightly grafts and re-transplanting them.

In the case where a botched surgery has resulted in bad skin exhibiting problems such as de-pigmentation, scarring or cobble stoning, there is a need for the skin to be repaired. This can be done by removing any abnormal scarring through excision and then smoothing the skin using dermabrasion or covering it up with follicular units to camouflage any remaining scars.

These are some of the ways you can have bad hair transplant results repaired. The thing to keep in mind is that there is no need for despair, and you don't have to live with the results of a bad transplant. There are many hair specialists available to correct any bad hair transplants.

Other Options Available

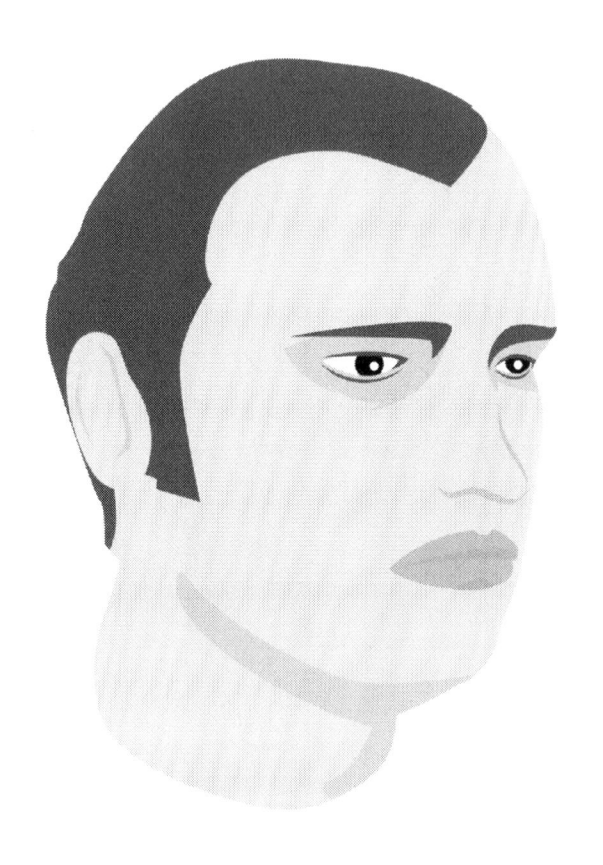

Scalp Micro-Pigmentation

This is a non-surgical form of hair grooming that can be used in place of a hair transplant in men and women. It involves the application of natural pigment onto the epidermis of the scalp to mimic real hair follicles. In short, it involves getting one's scalp tattooed with tiny marks that are similar to hair stubble, which will give you the appearance of having a buzz cut.

The advantage of undergoing this form of hair loss treatment is that there is no surgery involved and no scarring. This form of hair loss treatment works well for people who are dealing with complete hair loss. When you are bald, it is hard to get a hair transplant. First, there is no donor hair to use in a transplant and even if you decided to use synthetic hair it would cost a lot of money to graft it into the whole scalp. Plus there is the problem of the hair not looking natural and possibly falling out altogether.

Instead of risking these inconveniences, scalp pigmentation gives a ready solution that is neat and relatively painless, as compared to hair loss surgery, and gives patients the appearance of having some hair. This solution to hair loss can also be used to camouflage thinning hair. This is because the spaces can be tattooed using scalp pigmentation and these tattoos, in addition to the already present thinning hair, will give the impression of a full and thick head of hair.

Scalp pigmentation involves tattooing that does not penetrate the skin. The coloring agent used to make the tattoos can be matched to a person's hair color and skin tone, which ensures that the results look authentic. Many may be put off by the idea of using tattoo ink on their scalp. The good news is that this ink used in scalp pigmentation is a natural pigment that is not toxic. It also does not change color with time. If you choose black pigment, it will still be the same color a few years down the line.

This procedure is valued especially because the tattooing can be done in line with a patient's face shape, which will provide an overall attractive appearance. It costs less than a hair transplant, in some cases. This makes it a popular choice for anyone dealing with hair loss and thinning. The fact that it can be done for women as well as men makes it a popular choice.

As with all medical procedures, it is necessary to get an expert to do the procedure so that you are assured of good results. As there are bogus hair surgeons, you will also find bogus hair tattooing specialists that cannot be trusted to do a good job. So, before you settle for the right specialist, ensure that you get references that will assure you that he/she will do a good job. This kind of treatment is just another alternative to hair transplant surgery. It is excellent at treating hair loss and hair thinning without the patient having to use excessive amounts of money for the service or having to undergo painful surgery.

Hairline Lowering

This procedure is also known as forehead reduction. It is a surgery that is used to deal with a high hairline or a hairline that has receded excessively as a result of hair loss. This procedure is normally done on women, especially those of Chinese, Anglo–Saxon and East African origin who have a tendency to have high hairlines.

A low hairline can be caused by inadequate scalp laxity. It can also be a caused by trauma to the hair follicles as a result of traction alopecia. It is common for women to use harsh chemical treatments and undergo tight hair styles that end up uprooting the hair along the hairline. With time, the hairline ends up receding which results in a high hairline.

These issues can all be solved by having a hairline lowering procedure. It can also be used to deal with cases where one's hairline is in a shape that does not look attractive. In such a case, this procedure can be used to change a hairline to suit a person's face shape, thereby improving his/her appearance.

No matter the cause of a high hairline, there is no need to despair as hairline lowering can be used to solve the issue. This procedure involves the formation of a new hairline for an individual whereby the excess part of the forehead is cut off, and the scalp is stretched over to a point to achieve the desired hairline. The cut is done in such a way that hair will grow around the new hairline ensuring that it is undetectable.

While hair lowering surgery is a good option for many, it is often passed over in favor of hair grafting or hair transplants. This is because, in the case of hair transplants, there is no need to make an incision on the hairline. The use of hair transplants can make it easy for the surgeon to create an accurate hairline as hair is transplanted one graft after the other as opposed to hair lowering surgery where the surgeon has to struggle to shape a whole hairline.

However, for people that have a very high forehead the hair lowering technique can be used together with a hair transplant to achieve the desired results. In such a case, the forehead is first lowered and then the forehead shape is filled out using a minor hair transplant resulting in a full head of hair with a well-shaped hairline.

As in the case of hair transplants, hairline lowering requires a patient to use an expert doctor so that the desired results are achieved. When done properly, it can greatly improve one's hairline and lift an individual's self-esteem. Many women have used hair systems to deal with high foreheads, but if one needs a permanent solution to a high forehead, hair lowering is the answer.

It is just another helpful cosmetic technique available to help an individual achieve the kind of hairline that he/she desires. The fact that it can be done in conjunction with a hair transplant is an excellent advantage.

Eyebrow Restoration

Eyebrows are important facial features that help to improve one's appearance. It is common for women to be told that the state of their eyebrows will affect the way that they look. This is why procedures such as eyebrow plucking and tweezing are popular. They are used to shape one's eyebrows to suit the facial shape.

Unfortunately, women have overdone such eyebrow shaping techniques, which means that they end up without any eyebrows at all. Unlike in hair loss, the loss of eyebrows is perceived as an unnatural occurrence, and for this reason you will find people filling in their eyebrow regions by using eye pencils. Sometimes, the loss of eyebrows cannot be helped, such as in the case of burns, infections or a congenital inability to grow eyebrows.

Whatever the reason for eyebrow loss, an individual can deal with this problem by turning to eyebrow restoration. Eyebrow transplants cannot be compared to hair transplants. This is because the growth of the hair in the eyebrows cannot be compared to that of hair on the scalp. Eyebrow hair grows in different directions depending on its location in the eyebrow. The angle at which hair in the eyebrows grows is flat, which is in contrast to the angle of growth of hair on the scalp, which is 45 degrees.

Another aspect is that eyebrow hair grows in single strands while scalp hair follicles are composed of 1-4 hairs. The eyebrow growth cycle is quite short as these hairs only grow for 4 months in the Anagen phase, after which they shift to the Telogen phase and fall out. On the other hand, scalp hair can take as long as 3 – 7 years to complete a cycle. This is why hair from the scalp is used in eyebrow restoration.

Eyebrow restoration surgery ensures that eyebrows regain their fullness and in the case of thinning eyebrows, replaces them. It is also used to customize eyebrows where they do not grow or have been totally faced out due to trauma or excessive cosmetic procedures such as tweezing.

The donor hair used in this procedure is harvested from the scalp since as mentioned before these hairs have a long hair cycle and will continue to grow even after the transplant. The procedure involves transplanting the donor hair strands into small incisions. The incisions are cut in a right angle. This ensures that the transplanted hair strands follow the natural growth pattern typical to eyebrows.

An eyebrow transplant can use 50 – 325 hair strands depending on the extent of the hair loss and the density and size of hair needed. It is a short procedure that is quite painless and takes a short time to complete. After the procedure, there will be some scabbing and redness on the transplant region, but it fades as time goes by. Sutures are removed a week after the procedure. After this, the transplanted hair sheds two weeks later and re-grows after three months, after which it continues to grow for a lifetime.

Eyebrow hair transplants are quite valuable especially when restructuring eyebrows that have been lost due to burns and other forms of trauma.

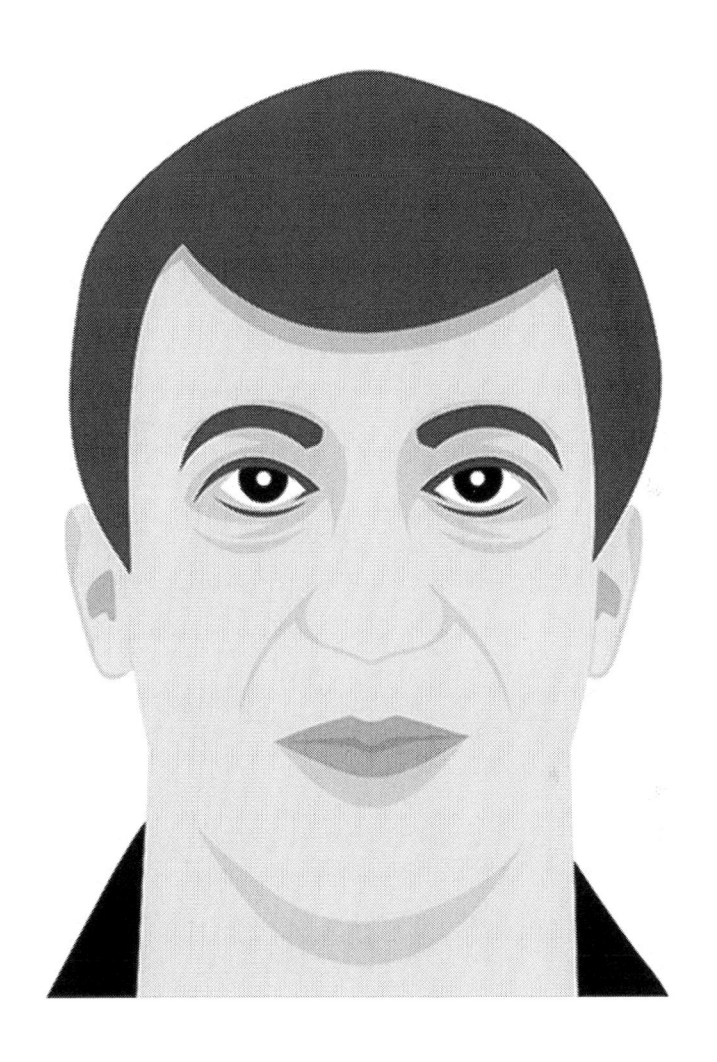

Printed in Great Britain
by Amazon